3D Echocardiography

Edited by

Takahiro Shiota MD FACC FESC
Professor of Medicine
Cleveland Clinic Lerner College of Medicine of the Case
Western Reserve University
Staff Cardiologist
Department of Cardiovascular Medicine
Cleveland Clinic
Cleveland, Ohio
USA

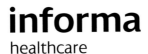

informa
healthcare

©2007 Informa UK Ltd

First published in the United Kingdom in 2007 by Informa Healthcare, Telephone House, 69-77 Paul Street, London EC2A 4LQ. Informa Healthcare is a trading division of Informa UK Ltd. Registered Office: 37/41 Mortimer Street, London W1T 3JH. Registered in England and Wales number 1072954.

Tel: +44 (0)20 7017 5000
Fax: +44 (0)20 7017 6699
Website: www.informahealthcare.com

Although every effort has been made to ensure that all owners of copyright material have been acknowledged in this publication, we would be glad to acknowledge in subsequent reprints or editions any omissions brought to our attention.

Although every effort has been made to ensure that drug doses and other information are presented accurately in this publication, the ultimate responsibility rests with the prescribing physician. Neither the publishers nor the authors can be held responsible for errors or for any consequences arising from the use of information contained herein. For detailed prescribing information or instructions on the use of any product or procedure discussed herein, please consult the prescribing information or instructional material issued by the manufacturer.

A CIP record for this book is available from the British Library.
Library of Congress Cataloging-in-Publication Data

Data available on application

ISBN-10: 1-84184-632-5
ISBN-13: 978-1-84184-632-3

Distributed in North and South America by
Taylor & Francis
6000 Broken Sound Parkway, NW, (Suite 300)
Boca Raton, FL 33487, USA

Within Continental USA
Tel: 1 (800) 272 7737; Fax: 1 (800) 374 3401
Outside Continental USA
Tel: (561) 994 0555; Fax: (561) 361 6018
Email: orders@crcpress.com

Distributed in the rest of the world by
Thomson Publishing Services
Cheriton House
North Way
Andover, Hampshire SP10 5BE, UK
Tel:+44 (0)1264 332424
Email: tps.tandfsalesorder@thomson.com

Composition by Exeter Premedia Services Private Ltd, Chennai, India
Printed and bound by Replika Press Pvt Ltd

Contents

Contributors

Philippe Acar MD PhD
Adult and Pediatric Congenital
Heart Disease Unit
Toulouse University Hospital
France

Fabrice Bauer MD
Head of Echocardiography
Cardiology Department
Hopital Charles Nicolle
Rouen Cedex
France

Hsuan-Hung Chuang MBBS M Med (Int Med) MRCP
Consultant Cardiologist
Department of Cardiology
National Heart Centre
Singapore

Erwan Donal MD
Echocardiography, Cardiology Department
Rennes University Hospital
France

K Gunasegaran MBBS M Med (Int Med)
Department of Cardiology
National Heart Center
Singapore

Takeshi Hozumi MD
Department of International Medicine and
    Cardiology
Osaka City University School of Medicine
Osaka
Japan

Luc J Jordaens MD PhD
Department of Cardiology
Thoraxcenter
Erasmus Medical Center
Rotterdam
The Netherlands

Jun Kwan MD
Department of Cardiology (Internal Medicine)
Inha University Hospital
Inchon
South Korea

Carles Paré MD PhD
Cardiology Department, Thorax Institute
Hospital Clinic
Barcelona
Spain

Jos RTC Roelandt MD PhD
Department of Cardiology
Thoraxcenter
Erasmus Medical Center
Rotterdam
The Netherlands

Florence Sheehan MD
Director, Cardiovascular Research and
    Training Center
University of Washington
Seattle, WA
USA

Takahiro Shiota MD FACC FESC
Professor of Medicine,
Cleveland Clinic Lerner College of Medicine
    of the Case
Western Reserve University
Staff Cardiologist
Department of Cardiovascular Medicine
Cleveland, Ohio
USA

Marta Sitges MD
Cardiology Department
Thorax Institute
Hospital Clinic
University of Barcelona
Spain

Asbjørn Stoylen MD
Department of Circulation and
Medical Imaging, Faculty of Medicine
Norwegian University of Science and Technology
Trondheim
Norway

Tamas Szili-Torok MD PhD
Department of Cardiology
Thoraxcenter
Erasmus Medical Center
Rotterdam
The Netherlands

Nozomi Watanabe MD
Department of Cardiology
Kawasaki Medical School
Kurashiki
Japan

Kiyoshi Yoshida MD
Department of Cardiology
Kawasaki Medical School
Kurashiki
Japan

Junichi Yoshikawa MD
President, Osaka Ekisaikai Hospital
Osaka
Japan

Preface

Echocardiography is now an indispensable tool in clinical cardiology. Quite a few textbooks are available at medical bookstores and on the internet where you can find new developing aspects of echocardiography. One of the most impressive and innovative advancements of echocardiography today is 3D echocardiography. There have been few comprehensive books to introduce this new echocardiographic method. Therefore, in this book, I would like to provide you with the most recent developments in this emerging field, focusing on the clinical values of 3D echocardiography.

For a long time now, 3D echocardiography has been recognized and conceived as an ideal tool for clinical cardiology. Three-dimensional ultrasound theoretically can provide what 2D echocardiography cannot; first, complete information about *absolute* heart chamber volumes, such as right ventricular volumes and aneurysmal left ventricular volumes. Second, 3D ultrasound also allows viewers an intuitive recognition of cardiac structures from any spatial point of view, such as *en face* views of the mitral valve leaflets. However, the idea had not materialized because of technical and engineering difficulties.

Quite recently, newer types of transthoracic real-time 3D echo systems have been developed, following the introduction of a real-time volumetric 3D system made by a small venture company in the mid-1990s. Nowadays, multiple powerful echo system vendors are engaged in this business with massive advertisements, which increasingly stimulate users' interests. The difference between the new models and older ones, including older type real-time 3D echo, is clear. First, the newer ones provide an easier, handier, and more user-friendly means to acquire and view 3D images. Second, image quality has improved significantly thanks to the advancement of ultrasound and computer technology.

Just a decade ago, it took almost a whole day to reconstruct a single 3D echocardiographic image with complicated gating and synchronization of many 2D planes. Those old-time 3D images were almost always miserable. Even after spending several hours putting the images together, it was hard to even find the location of the mitral valve. Now it takes only a few minutes to see 3D images of the mitral valve, seeing the heart as if you were a surgeon in the operating room. With the use of newer systems, you can at least tell the mitral anterior leaflet from the posterior leaflet, and when lucky, the location of the origin of the mitral regurgitation. You can visualize it thanks to the improved color Doppler 3D imaging of the most recent systems. Such blood flow information is quite valuable and is often indispensable in clinical cardiology.

Another important change in the clinical environment is the approval of reimbursement for 3D echocardiography in patients. Such advancement in technologic and socio-economic factors has prompted clinical application of this new technology. MRI and CAT can also provide us with 3D imaging even more impressively in certain patients, such as those with an aortic aneurysm. Still, 3D echocardiography shares some of the vital advantages that conventional 2D echocardiography has over the MRI/CAT scan: portability and handiness as well as Doppler color flow imaging.

As you will see in most chapters, there are still certain limitations to currently available 3D ultrasound methods, even with the help of state-of-the-art real-time 3D echo systems. In particular, relatively low image quality and low frame (volume) rate hinder everyday clinical use of 3D echocardiography. However, on-going strenuous efforts for further development of this method will overcome such limitations in the very near future. For example, real-time transesophageal 3D echocardiography which could provide stunning 3D valve motion images, was recently introduced in the literature and in clinical settings. Again, the fact remains that 3D echocardiography is one of the ultimate goals of cardiac imaging.

In this textbook, as this technology is still on the rise and not yet completed, we tried to demonstrate the *potential values* of 3D echocardiography in the everyday clinical setting of cardiology practice. In order to show the benefits of 3D echocardiography, some chapters show examples of conventional clinical 2D echocardiography with a hope to reveal the additive value of 3D information. Again, most chapters of this book are written for practical use while academically competent. Therefore, I did not intend to include massive, heavily complicated mathematic nor engineering aspects of 3D echocardiography for busy readers who are interested in the clinical applicability of this new method.

I sincerely hope that this textbook will provide you with essential knowledge and impressive pictures of modem 3D echocardiography for your practice in the twenty-first century.

Takahiro Shiota MD FACC FESC
Cleveland Clinic, Cleveland, Ohio, USA

Acknowledgments

The joys of making a book or a manuscript are many. The chief among them is acknowledging the assistance rendered by people who share the knowledge and the passion for finding innovative solutions to unsolved problems. I am grateful for the efforts made by all of the contributors who provided expert knowledge and quality 3D and 2D echocardiographic images.

I would like to express my thanks to the sonographers at the echo laboratory at Cleveland Clinic Heart Center, especially Hung Tran, RDCS, Debora A. Agler, RDCS, David A. Homa, RDCS, Helga P. Lombardo, RDCS, for acquiring excellent 3D echocardiographic images despite their busy daily clinical duties. I also would like to thank my associates, Drs Matsumura, Wada, Toyono, Yamano and Fukuda for their work on 3D rendering, reconstruction and analysis.

Furthermore, I wish to express my gratitude to Drs James D. Thomas, Mario J. Garcia and Richard A. Grimm for encouraging clinical applications of 3D echocardiography in the echo laboratory at the Department of Cardiovascular Medicine of Cleveland Clinic.

I am also indebted to the staff at Informa, especially Alan Burgess and Oliver Walter for tirelessly communicating with me and all the contributors, and Helen Brock for her careful editing and final preparation of this book.

Finally, I would like to give special thanks to my two daughters, Maiko Shiota, BS and Kanako Shiota, BA, for diligent proof reading and to my wife, Kinuko Shiota for her dedicated family support.

1 Evolution of Technology and Machine Basics

Hsuan-Hung Chuang and K Gunasegaran

INTRODUCTION

Among traditional screening techniques for quantitative assessment of cardiac function, including echocardiography, computed tomography (CT), nuclear imaging, and magnetic resonance imaging, echocardiography remains the fastest, least expensive, and least invasive screening modality. Over the last five decades the diagnostic capability of echocardiography has evolved dramatically from M-mode (1950s) to two-dimensional (2D) echocardiography (1970s). Whereas conventional 2D echocardiography is crucial to our understanding of the complex anatomy and 3D spatial relationships of cardiac structures, it requires the mental integration of a limited number of 2D imaging planes. This mental 3D reconstruction is inherently variable according to observer expertise, and can only be described to other clinicians or surgeons rather than displayed reproducibly. An actual 3D display format would provide a better insight into the functional and anatomic properties of cardiac structures and decrease variability both in the quality and the interpretation of complex pathology, among investigators.[1,2] The versatility of the 3D volumetric dataset allows clinicians to retrieve an infinite number of cross-sectional views, which permit more accurate and reproducible measurements of valve areas, masses, and cavity volumes by obviating geometric assumptions. The incorporation of new physiologic parameters will also provide additional information to address new clinical questions, such as left ventricular (LV) dyssynchrony in predicting potential benefits of cardiac resynchronization therapy for patients with congestive heart failure.

HISTORY AND DEVELOPMENT OF 3D ECHOCARDIOGRAPHY

The earliest ultrasound images were obtained using a single interrogation beam from a dedicated transducer. The ultrasound energy is sent out from the transducer as an ultrasound packet that is then reflected back to the transducer. Transmission of ultrasound from the transducer is not continuous but rather interrupted, with the non-transmit time being used to receive signals. The ultrasound along the single line of interrogation is reflected by cardiac structures and registered as a series of reflective interfaces. The location and strength of these interfaces can be plotted over time, yielding an M-mode echocardiography, which is accurate in the axial dimension only. While sampling rate may be high, information obtained from these images is extremely limited. 2D echocardiography, known for 30–40 years, provides an expanded view of cardiac anatomy by imaging not along a single line of interrogation, but along a series of lines typically spanning a 90° arc. Clinicians could visualize 2D orientation of the heart in both the axial and lateral dimensions. This together with the advent of Doppler and color Doppler added valuable information about the physiology and structure of the heart. However, it was no longer good enough to base decisions on mental conceptualization of a series of multiple orthogonal planar images into an imaginary multi-dimensional reconstruction, as this deduction was subjective.

Although 3D echocardiography has been part of the diagnostic landscape since the early 1970s, its evolution has been slow.[3] At the onset, its use was mainly confined to measurement of LV volumes using manual tracing methods from multiple cross-sectional views. These wire-frame views were very limited in their volumetric information yielded, and gave no additional information on the various structures within the heart and its hemodynamics. The early scanners were standalone machines, and devices were bulky and less maneuverable. The images were collected off-line, and then reconstructed and rendered to yield 3D images. Images were acquired mainly with transthoracic probes, which were attached to either motorized carriages or magnetic location sensors.[4,5] The image datasets were collected in linear, rotational, or fan-like manner, depending on the way in which the probe moved. Subsequent improvements in software and transducer technology allowed these 3D machines to collect data via the transesophageal route. The transesophageal studies often yielded greater clarity of the datasets, as compared to transthoracic studies.[6] Due to technical limitations, such as lack of processing power, relatively poor image quality, limited frame rates, and difficulties in image plane alignment, 3D echocardiography was very much limited to an experimental setting. The early 3D systems could not incorporate Doppler flow data, a critical aspect for diagnosis of flow through leaking valves and shunts.

Real-time 3D (RT3D) echocardiography and display were introduced in the late 1990s. Advances in the transducer technology, digital storage media, and software have made this imaging method clinically feasible. The newer generations of matrix-array transducers are able to capture pyramidal volumetric datasets of sufficient spatial and temporal resolution that can be rendered immediately to provide viewing and rapid interpretation. The new machines come with built-in software and hardware for 3D scanning so that there is no need for an additional stand-alone machine. It is now a clinical reality and a practical tool to perform RT3D echocardiography using transthoracic or transesophageal acoustic windows, in both adults and children.

PRINCIPLES OF 3D ECHOCARDIOGRAPHY

Historically, 3D echocardiography involved the compilation of multiple 2D images, where each image is defined with respect to its exact position in space. Technology has further evolved to make real-time imaging possible. Several different approaches have been used to acquire and reconstruct a 3D dataset. Though differing slightly, the fundamental steps can be divided into: data acquisition, data post-processing, and, lastly, image display and data analysis.

Data acquisition

Different equipment manufacturers have used different systems to obtain 3D imaging. There are essentially two basic approaches to data acquisition. The first method, called off-line 3D reconstruction, entails acquiring an entire sequence of images through either the transthoracic or transesophageal route, that is stored, processed externally by computer, and subsequently reconstructed into a 3D dataset. These 2D images are typically encoded with registration of the precise angle at which the heart is interrogated as well as electrocardiographic (ECG) and respiratory-gating information. The second and more promising method of 3D dataset acquisition is volumetric RT3D imaging.

Off-line 3D reconstruction

There are two approaches to off-line 3D reconstruction: random or sequential data acquisition. Random or freehand acquisition implies data collection being performed in a random order from different positions, and is essentially based on the free motion of the ultrasound transducer. Its advantage is that a series of cut-planes can be obtained from any available precordial acoustic window. This is accomplished by attachment of a mechanical arm to the transducer which, through either a series of position sensors or a spark gap or magnetic location device, determines the exact position and orientation of the transducer.[4,5,7] The transthoracic approach is used in this mode of acquisition. Surface-rendered or wire-frame reconstructions of selected structures are generated from manually or automatically derived contours in the cross-sectional images. This approach allows improved quantification of LV volume and mass, as the possibility of errors due to LV regional dysfunction or asymmetry is reduced.[8,9] One limitation is that the accurate endocardial border identification is restricted because of occasional big gaps between imaging planes. Reconstruction errors are also common due to the lack of synchronization between ECG and the scanner frame sampling. These pose problems in studying structures like cardiac valves and flow, as a high spatial and temporal resolution of images is important. In addition, a free-hand scanning system using the magnetic location device should not be used for patients with pacemakers who are pacemaker-dependent

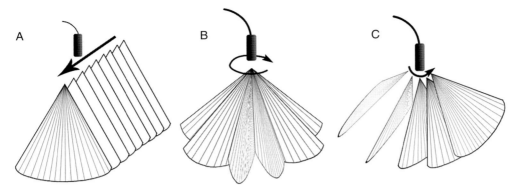

Figure 1.1 Different methods of sequential data acquisition for off-line 3D reconstruction. (A–C) Parallel scanning, rotational scanning, and fan-like scanning methods are shown from left to right.

because of the pulsed magnetic field generated by the magnetic transmitter. Because of the cumbersome nature of the free-hand scanning localization method and the complex nature of reconstruction, there has been little enthusiasm for this approach in clinical practice and it is currently not used.

A more common approach is sequential data acquisition.[10–12] Three different methods of sequential acquisition are possible with linear or parallel, fan-like, and rotational scanning (Figure 1.1). Either the transthoracic or the transesophageal approach can be adopted. The predetermined transducer movements are facilitated through various types of motorized carriage devices which are mounted with the transducer. These motors are controlled by the computer that is connected to the ultrasound machine. Rotational scanning is the most commonly employed method for acquiring images due to the relatively smaller acoustic window.

In the *linear or parallel scanning method*, the transducer, mounted on a motor assembly, translates perpendicularly to the imaging plane, linearly over the patient's surface in discrete, equal steps. This is similar to the scanning technique in CT. Parallel images are then stored and digitally combined to create a 3D dataset.[13] This method requires a large acoustic window and therefore is more suited for scanning the peripheral vessels, carotids, or abdominal structures, than the heart. Currently, this method is most often used in conjunction with intravascular ultrasound catheters.

With the *rotational scanning method*, a motor rotates the transducer array from 0 to 180° automatically at 3–5° increments around a fixed axis that is perpendicular to the array probe, creating a cone-shaped dataset and a 360° panoramic view of the cardiac structures.[14,15] The necessary acoustic window is only as big as the diameter of the transducer footprint. The transesophageal approach capitalizes on the rotational ability of the available multiplane transesophageal probe. The disadvantage is

the non-isotropic resolution of the dataset, with oversampling near the rotation axis and undersampling in the areas with a bigger radius from the middle axis. This needs to be compensated with interpolation techniques. Another inherent disadvantage is the middle artifact along the rotation axis. In addition, the rotational scan must always be complete (from 0 to 180°), otherwise the dataset cannot be used, because of missing structures in it.

With the *fan-like scanning method*, the mechanical assembly tilts the transducer about an axis parallel to the axis of the transducer. The image plane is swept in a fan, at regular angular intervals, to acquire a pyramidal or sector-shaped dataset. As for rotational scanning, a small echo window is theoretically sufficient. However, a small intercostal space could be a problem if the tilt angle is too big. Another disadvantage is that the color Doppler angle is dependent on the sweep angle, and therefore might not be constant as with parallel or rotational scanning. Unlike rotational scanning, the scanning process can be stopped if the target area is acquired.

As 2D images are acquired sequentially, respiratory and ECG gatings are necessary to account for motion artifacts caused by respiration and for registration of images in the time domain. After the ECG electrodes and the respiratory sensor have been placed on the patient, the 3D acquisition system analyzes the ECG R-wave to R-wave interval time and respiration signals for a learning period to calculate a representative heart cycle. The system defines the limits for acceptable heart cycles automatically and digitally records images of a complete heart cycle via gating logic. Alternatively, the user can interactively change or adapt these presets. Different sensor systems are currently used to register the patient's respiratory signal, either by sensing the impedance across the chest or measuring the temperature change via a nasal thermistor.

Volumetric RT3D echocardiography

The second and more promising method, also called volumetric imaging, is based on the design of a matrix phase-array transducer that instantaneously acquires a pyramidal volume dataset without complex post-processing. Prior to the advent of the matrix phase-array transducer, the sparse phase-array transducer was used for volumetric data acquisition. This transducer, consisting of 256 non-simultaneously firing elements, is capable of generating a pyramidal volume dataset within a single heartbeat. Images obtained can be displayed in two orthogonal (B-scan) and two to three parallel short-axis planes (C-scan).[1,16–18] However, the limitations include poor axial and lateral resolution, low operating frame rates, fixed narrow sector angle, and complicated off-line 3D rendering.

The full matrix phase-array transducer, first developed by von Ramm et al of Duke University, utilizes approximately 3000 elements (Figure 1.2).[1,19] These elements are arranged in a 2D grid, and using parallel processing techniques the matrix phase-array offers steering of the ultrasound beam in both the elevation and the azimuth plane. In contrast to the sparse array probe, the full matrix phase-array uses all its channels to transmit ultrasound pulses. This circumvents the fundamental limitation of the speed of ultrasound in the tissue as it is now possible to process several scan lines simultaneously. From the pyramidal volume, cross-sectional images at different depths can be selected on-line. This new transducer has improved side-lobe performance, higher sensitivity and penetration, and harmonic capabilities which may be used for both gray scale and contrast imaging. It also permits different modes of data acquisition, including narrow angle acquisition (60° × 30° pyramidal volumes), zoom mode (magnified view of a subsection of the pyramidal volume, 30° × 30° sector in high resolution), and wide-angled acquisition. The first two modes of data acquisition are predominantly used to visualize cardiac and valve morphology. The wide angled acquisition mode is often used to acquire the entire LV volume in order to perform detailed analysis of global and regional wall motion.

Volume-rendering algorithms are applied and gray-scale tissue information is available in the reconstructions, representing a significant advance over surface-rendered reconstructions. Overall, data acquisition is less time-consuming and less susceptible to artifacts. Although the newer machines do not need gating to respiration and ECG, a good ECG trace and regular breathing would certainly improve image dataset collection. The current generation of ultrasound does not have the computational power to acquire an entire 3D dataset in one cycle. For acquisition of a complete volume of cardiac data, four sequential cardiac cycles are typically

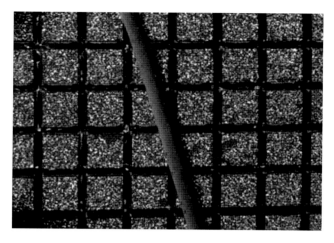

Figure 1.2 Microscopic view of a matrix phase-array transducer. Each small square is an active ultrasound element. The size of a human hair is shown for comparison. (Courtesy of Philips Medical Systems.)

captured and added to create a complete volume of information. In addition, the use of the matrix phase-array transducers also allows the option for simultaneous acquisition of true real-time biplane echocardiography in which any two planes can be simultaneously imaged.[20]

Data post-processing and rendering

Following data acquisition, the acquired 2D images are realigned, post-processed, and digitally reformatted into a Cartesian or 3D volumetric dataset. Depending on the acquisition method, different functions have to be used. Gaps or missing information between various sector-shaped beams in the acquired dataset must be filled using 3D interpolation algorithms. Image noise and motion artifacts created by patient or probe movement during the scan can be reduced or eliminated by special image processing filters and smoothing algorithms.

In order for subsequent analysis to be performed, the 3D volumetric dataset needs to be rendered or reconstructed within the ultrasound system. Volume-rendered reconstruction is a process whereby intracardiac structures are reconstructed within the computer memory so that the dataset can be sectioned electronically in any plane, allowing visualization of any structure within the heart from any viewpoint. By sectioning or cropping away parts of the dataset, it is possible to see inside the heart and view the anatomic orientation and motion of intracardiac structures. The 3D effect can be further enhanced by creating rotational sequences of the image upon display. Another method, called wire-frame or surface-rendered reconstruction, may be performed to produce an image with feature contours and depth perspective. Different algorithms and different shading techniques, such as texture shading, distance shading, and gradient shading, are used to define the segment of interest. Threshold limits are used to separate cardiac structures from the blood pool and background, and brightness and shading provide perception of depth. This approach allows for the assessment of characteristics such as structure and shape, and for improved quantification of LV volume.[7,11] More recently, 3D reconstruction has also been applied to the color Doppler information allowing a 3D representation of jets superimposed on the 3D gray scale image.

Image display and data analysis

There are basically two methods of displaying 3D datasets: (1) a 2D cross-sectional display from any desired cut-planes, or (2) a volume-rendered display. Using the intersecting gridlines that cut the 3D dataset, the 2D image along any of these interrogation gridlines can be viewed. Different standardizations (anyplane, paraplane, rotoplane, mainplane) of computer-generated 2D images have been demonstrated. In the anyplane mode, the examiner may generate 2D images in any desired cross-section of the heart, which can be physically unobtainable by conventional transthoracic or transesophageal acoustic windows. The paraplane mode provides a sequence of equidistant parallel cut-planes through a structure, which are then displayed all together. Images that are rotated around one middle axis, like images seen during rotation of the transducer, are provided by the rotoplane mode. Lastly the mainplane mode provides the best overview of a 3D structure through simultaneous display of three cut-planes that are orthogonal to each other. The availability and versatility using the volumetric dataset therefore permits the retrieval of an infinite number of cardiac cross-sections which allow more accurate and reproducible measurements of valve areas, masses, and cavity volumes by obviating geometric assumptions. The second method of display is to slice or crop the full-volume dataset to 'expose' the interior. This provides a 3D perspective of what is otherwise a 2D image (Figure 1.3). The most recent generation of RT3D echocardiogaphy can also acquire color Doppler information that can be processed in an identical manner.

There are two methods of data analysis: (1) morphologic or (2) quantitative analysis. Surface rendering of the endocardial border can create perspectives not achievable with conventional methods such as the *en face* view of atrial septal defects or the atrial view of the mitral valve. In complex congenital heart disease 3D echocardiography may provide better spatial orientation and easier communication with the cardiothoracic surgeons. Quantitative analysis of volumes, masses, and surfaces is only possible after manual contour tracing with several cut-planes generated from the 3D dataset. This procedure is time-consuming and limits use in clinical routine, even though validation studies demonstrated that 3D echocardiography determination of masses and volumes is superior to one- or two-dimensional techniques which are based on geometric assumptions.

The accurate non-invasive quantification of cardiac flow volumes is important in clinical cardiology. Though estimates of flow parameters can be

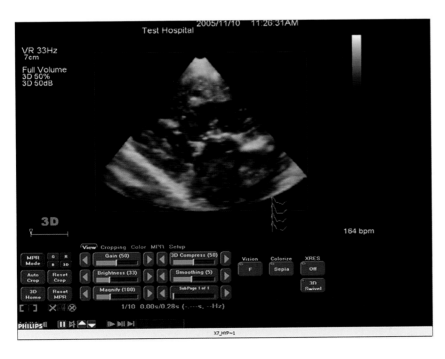

Figure 1.3 Real-time volumetric scan from transthoracic echocardiography. This full 3D dataset has been cropped so that the interior of the 3D volume has now been exposed. The versatility of the acquired 3D volumetric dataset permits the heart to be viewed or 'sliced open' in any imaging plane.

made by conventional 2D echocardiography, these methods may be unreliable when applied to complex, dynamic, 3D flow events.[21,22] The integration with color Doppler data and 3D flow quantification methods may lead to more precise quantification of valvular regurgitations. More recently, RT3D color Doppler echocardiography has been introduced. At present, frame rate, color Doppler quality, and clinical applications are still limited by the suboptimal acoustic sampling rate available for color Doppler.

LIMITATIONS OF CURRENT 3D TECHNOLOGY

Despite its unquestionable role in the diagnosis of heart disease and in the management of cardiac patients, 3D echocardiography does have some limitations, both in the morphologic visualization as well as in the functional assessment of the heart, such as blood flow, quantification of intracardiac volumes, etc. The prolonged acquisition time and tedious post-processing are important limiting factors that currently restrict routine clinical applications. One must also remember that the quality of 3D images is greatly dependent on the quality of 2D images, and thus the ability to obtain a motion- and artifact-free 3D dataset is critical. Possible inherent errors may be introduced by the off-line reconstruction technique, including spatial discordance due to movement of the heart, transducer, or patient during the acquisition process, and temporal discordance due to multiple beats needed for the rendered image. Although the newer RT3D machines utilize only 1–4 cardiac cycles to acquire and render images, the quality and accuracy of these images can still be affected by factors like irregular heart rhythms, tachycardia, and irregular breathing. If the acquisition is obtained via the transesophageal route, sedation of the patient is often necessary for this unpleasant procedure, with increased potential risks to the patient.

It must likewise be remembered that the basic image source for 3D echocardiography is the ultrasound wave. It is thus limited by the fundamentals of ultrasound waves. Since ultrasound waves are affected by signal loss from reflection, refraction, and attenuation, the image dataset obtained can be limited by these confounding factors, which can lead to areas of drop-out in the rendered images. In addition, certain structures which are highly echo-reflective, such as metallic prostheses, can cause acoustic shadowing which affects image quality. The acquisition angle of the transducer may not contain the entire structure of interest within the dataset, particularly in cases with dilated cardiac chambers. During the image reconstruction, the original gray value might be partially lost. On the other hand, operator-dependent changes in threshold settings, which define the tissue–blood interface on the 3D rendered display, can affect the apparent anatomic measurements. Measurements on reconstructed images should be made with caution, and the entire image post-reconstruction and interpretation thus requires a high degree of operator experience.[20]

ADVANCES AND FUTURE DEVELOPMENT

For several decades, no significant innovations have occurred at the level of the most basic determinants of ultrasound quality: the transducer elements or crystals that convert electrical into acoustic energy and vice versa. Piezoelectric crystal has been the cornerstone of the current ultrasound transducer. The coupling efficiency in converting electrical energy into pressure (sound) waves or vice versa is a key determinant of image quality. To create the overall piezoelectric effect, traditional piezoelectric crystals must be subjected to a poling process to align dipoles within polycrystalline materials. Due to the constraint of the grain boundaries of the piezoelectric crystals, only a fraction of dipoles can be aligned by an electric field and not all dipoles contribute to the acoustic response of the material. A recent breakthrough in improving the electro-mechanical coupling of the piezoelectric crystals, called PureWave crystals, has been introduced by Philips Medical System (Figure 1.4). These are more uniform and exhibit fewer defects, lower losses, and no grain boundaries. Boules or

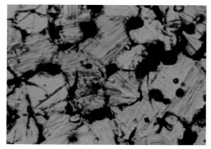

Imperfect, multi-crystalline, randomly orientated grains

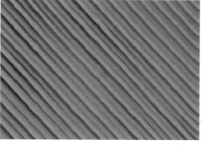

Perfect atomic level arrangement, uniform, no grain boundaries

Figure 1.4 The parallel lines showing in both piezoelectric and PureWave crystals are the ferroelectric domains. When the domains are properly aligned, they give better piezoelectric efficiency. (Courtesy of Philips Medical Systems.)

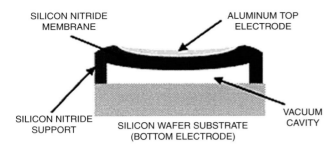

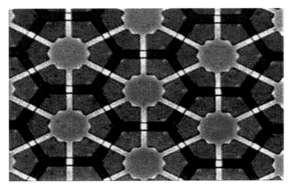

Figure 1.5 The upper panel illustrates silicon ultrasonic sensors which use drums built on the surface of the silicon to emit and receive ultrasound. The lower panel shows a portion of a silicon ultrasound transducer array. (Courtesy of Siemens Medical Solution.)

crystals are orientated along the desired crystallographic orientation(s) to maximize the crystal properties. When these crystals are poled at the preferred orientation(s), near perfect alignment of dipoles can be achieved, resulting in enhanced electro-mechanical properties. The efficiency of converting electrical to mechanical energy improves by as much as 68–85% compared to current piezoelectric ceramics. The PureWave crystals are reported to exhibit 10 times the strain compared to piezoelectric ceramics, enabling the achievement of significant gains in transducer bandwidth and sensitivity, and thus enhanced harmonic performance. This translates to improved ultrasound penetration and border delineation, and significantly reduced clutter with enhanced image resolution.

Another transducer innovation is the microelectromechanical systems technology developed by Sensant Corporation, which has since been acquired by Siemens Medical Solutions Ultrasound Division. These ultrasound transducers are made from silicon wafers using integrated circuit fabrication processes. Miniature 'drum heads', equivalent to one-seventh the cross-sectional size of a single strand of human hair, are formed from micro-fabricated silicon, with each drum operating as both an ultrasonic speaker and a microphone (Figure 1.5). The smaller the drum heads, the higher the frequency of the ultrasound signal. For pulse echocardiography, time-of-flight measurements, and Doppler fre-

quency shift detection, the higher frequency results in up to 10 times better timing and frequency resolution and up to a 10 times reduction of the dead zone. Unlike piezoelectric crystals, silicon transducers are nearly perfect unidirectional radiators that require no back damping materials and have no observable acoustic coupling with the sensor's supporting structure. These sensors, with a thickness of <1 mm, are typically much thinner than piezoelectric sensors for a given aperture size. The combination of a small form factor and an absence of mechanical coupling facilitates the design of small, less expensive systems. The tiny drum heads are particularly ideal for catheter transducers. In addition, the silicon sensors have a broader frequency response (200 kHz to 5 MHz) than most piezoelectric devices (50–2000 Hz). The improved bandwidth reduces signal ringing and signal distortion, thus improving the sensitivity. At present, single-element and 64-element one-dimensional arrays have been built for the medical imaging market. Multiple-element sensor arrays and sensor arrays with on-chip integrated electronics may be the next breakthrough for 3D imaging applications and in terms of manufacturing cost reduction. With multiple-element arrays, electronic beam steering or focusing is possible, as is off-axis beam radiation. Besides the tight integration of ultrasound beam-forming capabilities into the transducer, the new technology also enables the transducer, rather than the ultrasound system itself, to process the acquired data. The results are superior, yielding highly efficient volumetric RT3D imaging and higher image resolution. The integrated circuit technology streamlines the manufacturing process of transducers, making them more precise and flexible as well as increasing their quality.

Conventional ultrasound scanners utilize electronic transmitters and receivers at the scanner with a separate coaxial cable connected to each transducer element in the handle. The number of transducer elements determines the size and weight of the transducer cable assembly that connects the imaging array to the scanner. As the newer generation of matrix-array transducers allow new imaging modalities to be introduced, there is a significant increase in the channel count, making the transducer cable assembly more difficult to handle. Fiber optics can be used to transmit signals optically and has distinct advantages over the standard coaxial cable to increase flexibility and decrease the weight of the transducer cable for larger channel numbers.

What used to be the biggest limitation, the lack of real-time interaction, is now largely overcome by RT3D echocardiography. However, at present, 3D image rendering and reconstruction is fairly operator-dependent. In the future, improved tissue characterization with automated quantification, similar to CT, and matrix array probes that allow wider angled acquisition will make the operator's tasks easier. The ability to image a single cardiac cycle will obviate the need for gating to electrocardiography and respiration. Leading software companies are coming up with processing and reconstruction solutions with unprecedented speed for the next generation ultrasound scanners. 3D visualization and analysis software can be run on high-end personal computers to provide clinically proven applications, such as mitral valve analysis, LV dyssynchrony study, right ventricular analysis, etc.

CONCLUSION

Though 3D echocardiography is a technique that is still in evolution, it is no longer a cumbersome tool which is time-consuming to do or requires a lot of steps to get started. Advances in ultrasound technology have improved the speed, reproducibility, and accuracy of echocardiographic data captured. Continuing improvements in computing power

and sophistication have led to the development of 3D workstations, which can process 3D datasets in a matter of seconds to minutes. Integration of software into the ultrasound machine will also permit online processing of data. The eventual goal is RT3D display of cardiac anatomy, incorporating modalities such as Doppler flow and tissue imaging, M-mode echocardiography, and contrast echocardiogaphy. The accuracy of 3D echocardiography in providing a more authentic representation of cardiac morphology and calculation of flow, volume, and mass will greatly enhance the diagnostic confidence of echocardiography, and benefit the interventionist, the surgeon, and ultimately, the patient.

ACKNOWLEDGMENTS

The authors would like to acknowledge Philips Medical Systems and Siemens Medical Solution for the reproduction of images.

REFERENCES

1. Sheikh K, Smith SW, von Ramm O, Kisslo J. Real-time, three-dimensional echocardiography: feasibility and initial use. Echocardiography 1991; 8: 119–25.

2. De Castro S, Yao J, Pandian NG. Three-dimensional echocardiography: clinical relevance and application. Am J Cardiol 1998; 81: 96–102G.

3. Lange A, Palka P, Burstow DJ, Godman MJ. Three-dimensional echocardiography: historical development and current applications. J Am Soc Echocardiogr 2001; 14: 403–12.

4. Gopal AS, Keller AM, Rigling R, King DL Jr, King DL. Left ventricular volume and endocardial surface area by three-dimensional echocardiography: comparison with two-dimensional echocardiography and nuclear magnetic resonance imaging in normal subjects. J Am Coll Cardiol 1993; 22: 258–70.

5. Sapin PM, Schroder KM, Gopal AS et al. Comparison of two- and three-dimensional echocardiography with cineventriculography for measurement of left ventricular volume in patients. J Am Coll Cardiol 1994; 24: 1054–63.

6. Hozumi T, Yoshikawa J. Three-dimensional echocardiography using a multiplane transesophageal probe: the clinical applications. Echocardiography 2000; 17: 757–64.

7. King DL, Harrison MR, King DL Jr et al. Improved reproducibility of left atrial and left ventricular measurements by guided three-dimensional echocardiography. J Am Coll Cardiol 1992; 20: 1238–45.

8. Gopal AS, Schnellbaecher MJ, Shen Z et al. Freehand three-dimensional echocardiography for determination of left ventricular volume and mass in patients with abnormal ventricles: comparison with magnetic resonance imaging. J Am Soc Echocardiogr 1997; 10: 853–61.

9. Sapin PM, Gopal AS, Clarke GB, Smith MD, King DL. Three-dimensional echocardiography compared to two-dimensional echocardiography for measurement of left ventricular mass anatomic validation in an open chest canine model. Am J Hypertens 1996; 9: 467–74.

10. Ludomirsky A, Vermilion R, Nesser J et al. Transthoracic real-time three-dimensional echocardiography using the rotational scanning approach for data acquisition. Echocardiography 1994; 11: 599–606.

11. Pandian NG, Roelandt J, Nanda NC et al. Dynamic three-dimensional echocardiography: methods and clinical potential. Echocardiography 1994; 11: 237–59.

12. Roelandt J, Salustri A, Mumm B, Vletter W. Precordial three-dimensional echocardiography with a rotational imaging probe: methods and initial clinical experience. Echocardiography 1995; 12: 243–52.

13. Binder T, Globits S, Zangeneh M et al. Three-dimensional echocardiography using a transoesophageal imaging probe. Potentials and technical considerations. Eur Heart J 1996; 17: 619–28.

14. Roelandt JR. Three-dimensional echocardiography: new views from old windows. Br Heart J 1995; 74: 4–6.

15. Yao J, Cao QL, Pandian NG et al. Multiplane transthoracic echocardiography: image orientation, anatomic correlation, and clinical experience with a prototype phased array multiplane surface probe. Echocardiography 1997; 14: 559–78.

16. Ahmad M, Xie T, McCulloch M, Abreo G, Runge M. Real-time three-dimensional dobutamine stress echocardiography in assessment stress echocardiography in assessment of ischemia: comparison with two-dimensional dobutamine stress echocardiography. J Am Coll Cardiol 2001; 37: 1303–9.

17. Shiota T, McCarthy PM, White RD et al. Initial clinical experience of real-time three-dimensional echocardiography

in patients with ischemic and idiopathic dilated cardiomyopathy. Am J Cardiol 1999; 84: 1068–73.

18. von Ramm OT, Smith SW. Real time volumetric ultrasound imaging system. J Digit Imaging 1990; 3: 261–6.

19. Kisslo J, Firek B, Ota T et al. Real-time volumetric echocardiography: the technology and the possibilities. Echocardiography 2000; 17: 773–9.

20. Binder TM, Moertl D, Mundigler G et al. Stereolithographic biomodeling to create tangible hard copies of cardiac structures from echocardiographic data: in vitro and in vivo validation. J Am Coll Cardiol 2000; 35: 230–7.

21. Miyatake K, Izumi S, Okamoto M et al. Semiquantitative grading of severity of mitral regurgitation by real-time two-dimensional Doppler flow imaging technique. J Am Coll Cardiol 1986; 7: 82–8.

22. Helmcke F, Nanda NC, Hsiung MC et al. Color Doppler assessment of mitral regurgitation with orthogonal planes. Circulation 1987; 75: 175–83.

2 Left Ventricle

Takeshi Hozumi and Junichi Yoshikawa

TWO-DIMENSIONAL ECHOCARDIOGRAPHY

Left ventricular (LV) dimensions, volume, and wall thickness obtained from echocardiography are widely used indices in clinical practice and trials.[1] Although visual assessment of LV size and systolic function is frequently used, it depends on the observer's skill. Thus, quantification of LV size, systolic function, and mass using two-dimensional (2D) echocardiography has been recommended; the methods have been validated in earlier studies.[2–5]

LV volume

In patients with wall motion abnormalities, LV volume and ejection fraction (EF) are especially important as prognostic predictors and physiologic indices.[6,7] LV volume and EF from linear dimensions from 2D images using the methods of Teichholz or Quinones may be inaccurate because they are based on geometric assumptions.[8,9] The most commonly used method for volume measurement recommended by the American Society of Echocardiography is the biplane method of disks (modified Simpson's rule) (Figure 2.1).[10] Because this 2D method minimizes mathematic assumptions, more accurate values of LV volume and EF can be obtained compared with the Teichholz or Quinones methods from LV linear dimensions. The principle of this method is that the total LV volume can be calculated from the summation of elliptical disks. However, 2D methods still have technical limitations for LV volume measurement in patients with LV asynergy, especially with LV distortion. Underestimation of LV volume has been reported compared with angiography or magnetic resonance imaging (MRI).[11–14] Errors in image plane positioning may be the most important problem in 2D echocardiography for the LV volume estimation. The apex is frequently foreshortened in the apical views because of difficulty in obtaining an adequate apical echocardiographic window in most patients.[11] Another limitation of 2D methods is that 2D echocardiography still has geometric assumptions because it can evaluate only four walls of the LV (anterior, inferior, lateral, and septum), and wall motion abnormalities in the anteroseptum, and posterior walls cannot be evaluated in the recommended biplane method. In addition, significant operator (different sonographers) and observer (different reading doctors) variabilities may be another limitation of 2D echocardiography, especially in serial studies.

LV mass

LV hypertrophy is a strong predictor of cardiovascular morbidity and mortality in patients with essential hypertension[15,16] and coronary artery disease.[17,18] Furthermore, LV mass offers better prognostic information, facilitating identification of individuals at high risk of stroke and transient ischemic attack.[19] Thus, an accurate and reproducible non-invasive method for determining LV mass in individual patients is an important advance in clinical cardiology.

LV mass has been calculated using linear measurements from the LV diameter and wall thickness.[20] The formula for estimation of LV mass from LV linear dimensions can only be used in patients without distortions of LV geometry from the following formula: please note LVIDd = left ventricular diameter at end-diastole

$$LV\ mass = 0.8 \times \{1.04[(LVIDd + PWTd + SWTd)3 - (LVIDd)3]\} + 0.6\ g$$

where PWTd and SWTd are posterior and septal wall thicknesses at end-diastole, respectively.

The most commonly used 2D methods for measuring LV mass are based on the area–length formula and the truncated ellipsoid model, as described in the 1989 ASE recommendation on LV

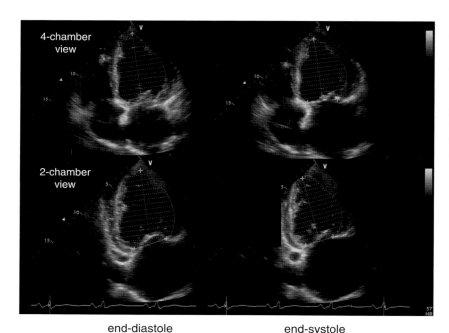

Figure 2.1 LV volume measurement by 2D echocardiography. In 2D echocardiography, LV volumes can be calculated from apical 4-chamber (upper) and 2-chamber cross-sections (lower) by the summation of disks method. For LV volume calculation, the LV endocardial border in both cross-sections is traced at end-diastole (left) and end-systole (right).

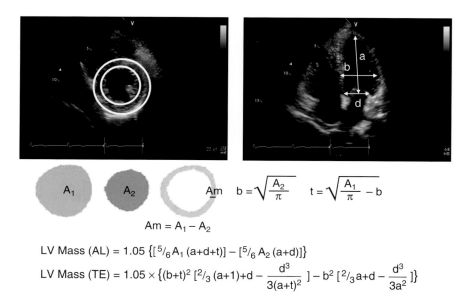

$$Am = A_1 - A_2$$

$$b = \sqrt{\frac{A_2}{\pi}} \qquad t = \sqrt{\frac{A_1}{\pi}} - b$$

$$\text{LV Mass (AL)} = 1.05 \left\{ \left[\tfrac{5}{6} A_1 (a+d+t) \right] - \left[\tfrac{5}{6} A_2 (a+d) \right] \right\}$$

$$\text{LV Mass (TE)} = 1.05 \times \left\{ (b+t)^2 \left[\tfrac{2}{3} (a+1) + d - \frac{d^3}{3(a+t)^2} \right] - b^2 \left[\tfrac{2}{3} a + d - \frac{d^3}{3a^2} \right] \right\}$$

Figure 2.2 LV mass measurement by 2D echocardiography. In 2D echocardiography, LV mass can be calculated from the short-axis (left) and apical 4-chamber cross-sections (right) by one of the two formulas as shown in this figure; upper formula: area–length method (AL), lower formula: truncated ellipsoid method (TE), where A_1 = total LV area; A_2 = LV cavity area, Am = myocardial area, a is the long or semi-major axis from the widest minor axis radius to the apex, b is the short-axis radius, and d is the truncated semi-major axis from the widest short-axis diameter to the mitral annulus plane. Assuming a circular area, the radius (b) is computed and mean wall thickness (t) derived from the short-axis epicardial and cavity areas. A_1 = area including LV myocardium and LV intracavity, A_2 = LV intracavity area, A_m = LV myocardial area.

quantitation.[21] LV mass can be calculated by one of the two formulas shown in Figure 2.2. The accuracy and reproducibility of 2D echocardiography for LV mass measurement are moderately improved over those of linear dimensions methods,[22,23] although increased difficulty in obtaining suitable quality images may limit the ability to determine LV mass. In addition, 2D echocardiography is still limited by the need for assumptions about ventricular shape.[24]

These uncertainties limit the effectiveness of clinical echocardiography for assessing changes of LV mass over serial studies.

THREE-DIMENSIONAL ECHOCARDIOGRAPHY

3D volume measurement requires no geometric assumptions, even in patients with wall motion abnormalities. Thus, 3D echocardiography is potentially an ideal tool for determining LV volume, EF, and LV mass, even in patients with wall motion abnormalities. Several 3D echocardiographic techniques have been developed and applied to LV volume[25–55] and mass[55–61] determination during the last decade. 3D techniques can be divided mainly into two types: (1) a reconstruction technique which needs data acquisition of multiple 2D images and (2) a real-time technique which provides volumetric image data acquisition.

LV volume

Reconstruction techniques for 3D echocardiography

In earlier studies the reconstruction method of 3D data acquisition was used, in which multiple 2D images are collected by free-hand scanning[25–32] or gated sequential scanning.[33–37,46–49]

Free-hand scanning For free-hand scanning, the 3D echocardiographic system, which consists of an acoustic spatial locater or spark gap and personal computer, is linked to a conventional 2D echocardiographic machine.[25–32] LV 3D data are computed from 7 to 10 short-axis 2D images acquired with a line-of-intersection display as a guide. This display is created by the parasternal long-axis cross-section, which serves as the reference image. The short-axis cross-sections are spaced from the inferior surface of the aortic valve throughout the body of the left ventricle to the apex. All images for 3D reconstruction are acquired during suspended respiration. 3D images are reconstructed at both end-diastole and end-systole for LV volume calculation. 3D LV volume is computed from the traced endocardial boundaries of each short-axis section at both end-diastole and end-systole using a polyhedral surface reconstruction algorithm. It has been reported that LV volume and ejection fraction obtained by 3D echocardiography with the free-hand scanning method are more accurate and have less variability than those obtained by 2D echocardiography, when using MRI or radionuclide angiography as the gold standard for comparison. However, time required for acquisition of each dataset is at least 6–8 minutes in this method. In cases with difficulty of data acquisition, it may be prolonged.

Gated sequential scanning In *rotational scanning* (Figure 2.3) by the transthoracic approach, an external stepper motorized device is attached to a commercially available transducer, while the conventional 2D echocardiographic system is interfaced with a 3D reconstruction computer system. Sequential cross-sectional images are acquired at 2–5° steps from the apical transducer position, under the gating of ECG and respiration. The multiplane

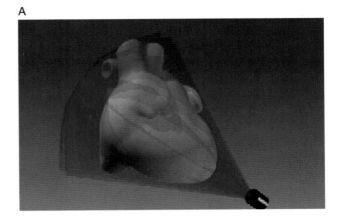

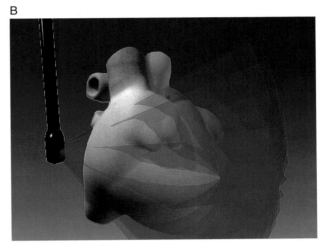

Figure 2.3 3D echocardiography by rotational scanning. In the transthoracic approach, multiple cross-sections are acquired by rotating the transducer (A). In the transesophageal approach, the multiplane transducer provides multiple cross-sections without changing the position of the probe (B).

transesophageal echocardiography (TEE) probe is used for rotational scanning with or without a rotational device. For acquisition of 3D image data, the TEE probe is positioned at the mid-esophageal portion, and is kept stationary during data acquisition. The scanning plane of the heart is obtained by rotating the transducer at 2–5° angular increments around a 180° arc, starting from a 4-chamber view using ECG and respiratory gating. Once the scanning sequence is completed, the digital images are stored in the memory and formatted in a cubic dataset of the entire cardiac anatomy over one cardiac cycle in both the transthoracic and transesophageal approach. It has been reported that LV volume and ejection fraction from the 3D approach using multiplane TEE correlated highly with those obtained by cineventriculography.[35] Average image acquisition time is 5 to 10 minutes in rotational scanning. The 3D approach with multiplane TEE can be used especially in intraoperative evaluation.

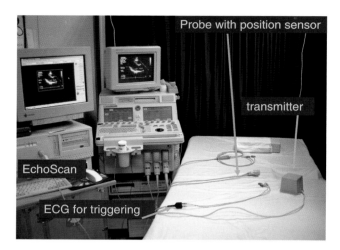

Figure 2.4 3D echocardiography by free-hand gated sequential scanning using a magnetic tracking device.

The free-hand gated sequential scanning system using a magnetic tracking device (Figure 2.4) consists of a position sensor, a receiver, and a personal computer for 3D reconstruction. These systems are linked to the conventional 2D ultrasound system with the same transducer. Transducer position and orientation are recorded with a magnetic tracking system. The position sensor is rigidly attached to the echocardiographic transducer. Before the actual image acquisition, the R–R intervals are predetermined with an acceptable variability of 150 ms or less and respiration is gated at the end-expiratory phase. On the basis of this information, the cross-sectional images are acquired during the entire cardiac cycle. The images are acquired from the apical views, and 6–9 consecutive sections are then recorded with 20–30° intervals by manual rotation of the transducer (Figure 2.5). The time-varying dipole x, y, and z electromagnetic fields generated by the position sensor are detected by the receiver. The images are digitally stored in the personal computer, and end-diastolic and end-systolic endocardial borders are manually traced in 6–9 apical images from the stored image data. Computer-generated 3D reconstruction of the LV cavity is performed, and end-diastolic volume, end-systolic volume, and EF are calculated by average rotational geometry. Figure 2.6 shows an example of the 3D LV endocardial surface reconstructed in free-hand gated sequential scanning in a patient without segmental wall motion abnormality. Although accurate LV volume measurement by the reconstruction method has been demonstrated in the previous reports, there is a time limitation in the process – this method requires 3–10 minutes for 3D data acquisition, even under ideal conditions. Prolonged acquisition times increase the chance of patient motion or artifacts, resulting in unsuccessful 3D image reconstruction.

Real-time technique for 3D echocardiography

The real-time (RT) volumetric method, which requires only one cycle for 3D data acquisition, has overcome the problem of prolonged acquisition time. The first generation of RT3D systems had a matrix-array transducer with 256 elements attached to the special machine for 3D echocardiography. A $60° \times 60°$ pyramidal volume dataset could be acquired in a single heart beat by this system. However, 3D images were not displayed in real time, and only several 2D images were displayed simultaneously in this system. Several studies have reported that the values for LV volume and EF obtained from the first-generation systems had a good correlation with those obtained from MRI[42–44] and multigated radionuclide angiography.[45] However, the image quality of first-generation RT3D echocardiography was comparatively poor because of relatively low spatial resolution.[40,42]

The introduction of the new generation of RT3D echocardiography has provided an easy process for both 3D data acquisition and 3D LV volume analysis with good image quality in a standard ultrasound machine. In the new RT3D echocardiography, the newly developed matrix-array transducer uses 3000 active elements for real-time 3D imaging, giving improved image quality. 3D images of $15° \times 60°$ pyramidal volume can be demonstrated in real time by this new 3D system. To acquire the entire LV data for volume analysis, four sectors of about $15° \times 60°$ should be scanned during four consecutive heart beats. The apical approach is generally used to acquire full volumetric datasets of the left ventricle. After visualizing apical 4- or 2-chamber views as reference images using 2D echocardiography, full-volume volumetric datasets are acquired, during four consecutive heart beats, without moving the transducer. The four subvolumes are automatically integrated and the entire pyramidal approximately $80° \times 80°$ dataset is obtained for acquisition of full LV volume (Figure 2.7). The LV full volume datasets are stored on optical disks and can be transferred to a personal computer. End-diastolic volume, end-systolic volume, and EF are calculated, usually by the average rotation method with 4–8 apical cross-sectional images, using LV volume measurement software. The endocardial border of the left ventricle is manually (Figure 2.8) or semi-automatedly (Figure 2.9) traced in each cross-sectional image at end-diastole and end-systole. Finally, the entire 3D LV intracavity is reconstructed (Figure 2.9), and the LV end-diastolic and end-systolic volumes and LV EF are calculated by the computer software.

Excellent correlations regarding LV volume and EF have been reported when the 3D method is compared with the radionuclide method (quantitative gated single-photon emission CT, QGS)[51]

A
B
C

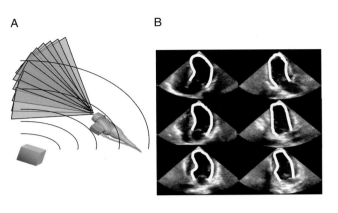

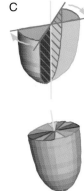

Figure 2.5 Free-hand gated sequential scanning using a magnetic tracking device. (A) The magnetic tracking system and receiver. The receiver is glued to the ultrasound probe. The time-varying dipole x, y and z electromagnetic fields generated by the position sensor are detected by the receiver. (B) Traced LV endocardial borders from apical 6 images. (C) Reconstruction of LV cavity using average rotation method.

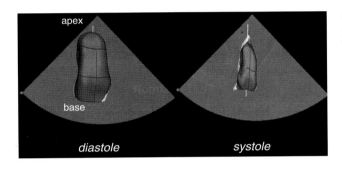

Figure 2.6 LV shape demonstrated by 3D echocardiography with free-hand gated sequential scanning in a patient without segmental wall motion abnormality.

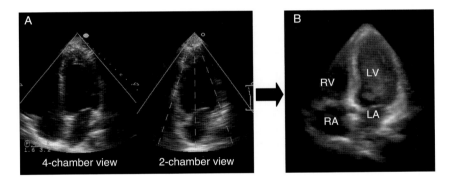

Figure 2.7 Acquisition of full LV volume by new real-time 3D (RT3D) echocardiography. After visualizing the 4-chamber view as a reference image, 4 sectors of 20° × 80° are scanned during 4 heart beats without moving the transducer (A). The four subvolumes are automatically integrated, and the entire pyramidal approximately 80° × 80° dataset is obtained for acquisition of full LV volume. (B) RT3D image cropped to the 4-chamber view, obtained from full volume 3D data.

and with MRI.[52] A study evaluating LV volume by the new RT3D method in patients with asynergy due to coronary artery disease[51] showed that it correlated well with the radionuclide method in the measurement of LV volume (Figure 2.10). It also correlated well with the radionuclide method in the measurement of both end-diastolic and end-systolic volume ($r = 0.97$, mean difference = 3.4 ± 14.0 ml and $r = 0.98$, mean difference = 2.0 ± 8.7 ml, respectively), while 2D echocardiography also correlated with the radionuclide method in the

measurement of both end-diastolic volume and end-systolic volume, but underestimated LV volume ($r = 0.98$, mean difference = 21.1 ± 20.7 ml and $r = 0.98$, mean difference = 15.6 ± 17.1 ml, respectively) (Figure 2.10(A) and (B)). EF obtained by real-time 3D echocardiography had better agreement with that obtained by the radionuclide method than that obtained by 2D echocardiography ($r = 0.92$, mean difference = −0.2 ± 4.6% and $r = 0.89$, mean difference = −2.7 ± 5.8%, respectively) (Figure 2. 10(C)). With the RT3D echocardiography,

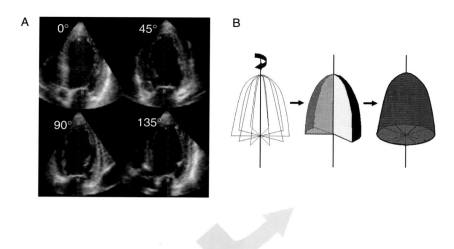

Figure 2.8 LV volume calculation by real-time 3D echocardiography using the average rotation method. The endocardial border of the left ventricle is traced in each cross-sectional image (0°, 45°, 90°, 135°) at end-diastole and end-systole (A). LV volume is calculated (B).

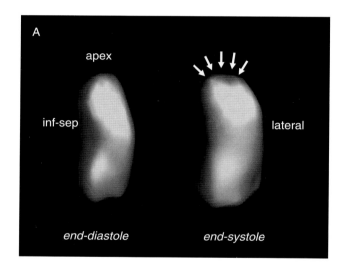

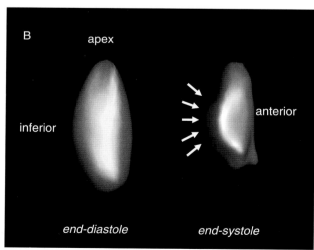

Figure 2.9 LV shape demonstrated by new real-time 3D echocardiography. (A) The reconstructed LV cavity in a patient with wall motion abnormality in the apical wall (left: end-diastole, right: end-systole). (B) The reconstructed LV cavity in a patient with wall motion abnormality in the inferior wall (left: end-diastole, right: end-systole). Inf-sep=inferior septum.

intra- and interobserver variabilities for end-diastolic volume, end-systolic volume, and EF were 4.0% and 5.9%, 6.1% and 7.0%, and 4.7% and 5.0%, respectively.[51] This suggests that this method may be useful in the measurement of LV function in the clinical setting.

Another similar study also reported that new RT3D echocardiography also allows us to measure accurate LV volume and EF comparative to cardiac MRI.[52] More accurate estimations of LV volume and EF were achieved with new RT3D echocardiography than with 2D echocardiography. 3D LV volume measurements were highly reproducible in both studies. Compared with magnetic resonance data, LV volumes calculated from 3D echocardiography showed significantly better agreement (smaller bias), lower scatter, and lower intra- and interobserver variability than 2D echocardiography.[52] Regarding the feasibility of new RT3D echocardiography, only 2 of 28 (7%) patients with wall motion abnormalities in the report were excluded from the study because of inadequate RT3D echocardiography images.[51] In the other recent study, similar feasibilities were shown.[52]

LV volume analysis by 3D echocardiography

The summation of disks method (Figure 2.11) allows accurate quantification of LV volume and EF, and has been utilized in previous studies. In this method, LV endocardial tracing in multiple short-axis cross-sections from base to apex is required at both end-diastole and end-systole for calculation of LV end-diastolic and end-systolic volumes, and LV EF. The accuracy reduces with decreasing number of short-axis cross-sections, particularly in patients with wall motion abnormalities.[36] Thus, the major problem of the summation of disks method for clinical application is the time-consuming

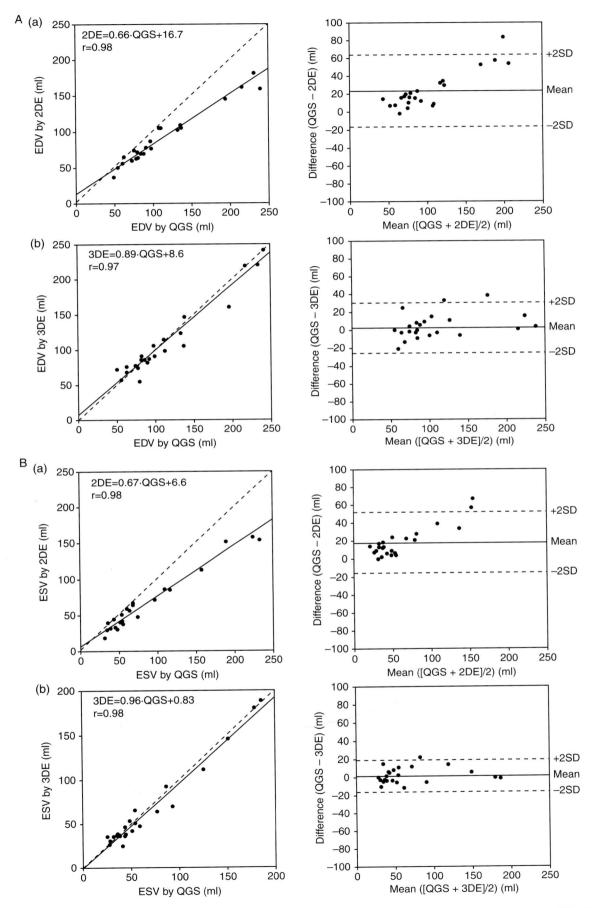

(*Continued*)

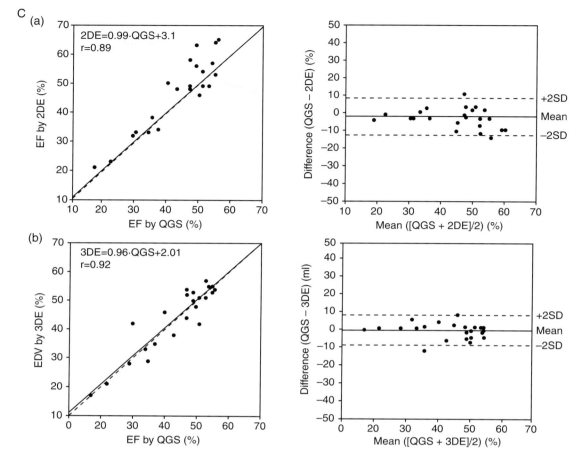

C (a)

2DE=0.99·QGS+3.1
r=0.89

EF by 2DE (%)

EF by QGS (%)

Difference (QGS – 2DE) (%)

+2SD
Mean
–2SD

Mean ([QGS + 2DE]/2) (%)

(b)

3DE=0.96·QGS+2.01
r=0.92

EDV by 3DE (%)

EF by QGS (%)

Difference (QGS – 3DE) (ml)

+2SD
Mean
–2SD

Mean ([QGS + 3DE]/2) (%)

Figure 2.10   LV end-diastolic volume (A), end-systolic volume (B), and ejection fraction (C) by new real-time 3D (RT3D) echocardiography. a) Regression analysis (left) and mean difference ± 2SD (right) between quantitative gated SPECT (QGS) and 2D echocardiography (2DE) for end-diastolic volume (EDV), end-systolic volume (ESV), and ejection fraction (EF). b) Regression analysis (left) and mean difference ± 2SD (right) between QGS and RT3D echocardiography (3DE) for EDV, ESV, and EF.

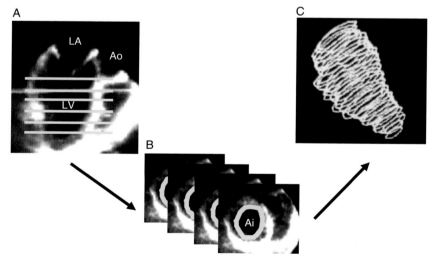

A

LA
Ao
LV

B

Ai

C

Figure 2.11   Calculation of LV volume using the summation of disks methods in 3D echocardiography. (A) In the long-axis cross-sectional views reconstructed from the cubic dataset, the level of the short-axis cross-section was determined by the line shown in the figure. (B) The endocardial border is traced in each short-axis cross-sectional view at end-diastole or end-systole. (C) Wire frame model of the left ventricle at end-diastole or end-systole is demonstrated after the summation of tracing of the LV endocardial border in every short-axis cross-section. LV = left ventricle, LA = left atrium, A0 = aorta, Ai = LV intracavity area.

process of endocardial tracing. On the other hand, the average rotation method (Figure 2.8) demands fewer component image planes than the summation of disks method for 3D measurement of LV volume and EF. It was shown that the time required for the determination of LV volume and EF was shorter using the average rotation method than the summation of disks method.[60] However, LV endocardial manual tracing or semi-automated tracing with manual correction is still a time-consuming

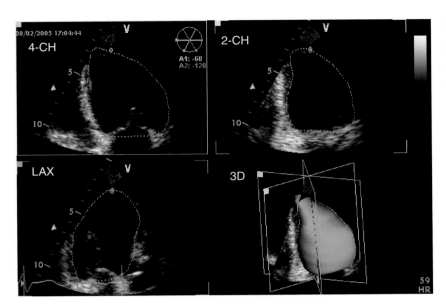

Figure 2.12 Triplane demonstration in real-time 3D echocardiography. By tracing the LV endocardium in the 4-chamber (4-CH), 2-chamber (2-CH), and long-axis (LAX) views, a 3D LV endocardial shape is reconstructed and LV volume can be calculated.

process in clinical echocardiography. The triplane method may be practical for routine echocardiography in patients without LV asynergy in the antero-lateral and infero-septum walls because this method requires LV endocardial tracing in only three cross-sections (Figure 2.12).

Recently developed semi-automated LV volume analysis software provides a quick calculation of 3D LV volume.[54] First, anatomically correct apical 2- and 4-chamber views at end-diastole are extracted from the pyramidal dataset on the first frame in the loop (Figure 2.12(A)). Then five anatomic landmarks are manually initialized: two points to identify the mitral valve annulus in the two apical views and one point for the apex. Then the same procedure is performed in the frame at end-systole. Following manual identification of these points, the program automatically identifies the 3D endocardial surface. Finally, LV end-diastolic volume, end-systolic volume, and EF are automatically calculated (Figure 2.12(B)). Not only a time–entire LV volume curve but also a time–segmental LV volume can be demonstrated from the 3D dataset (Figure 2.14). These individual curves, representing segmental wall motions, can be used for the assessment of LV dyssynchrony.

LV mass

LV mass measurement by RT3D echocardiography[52,56–62]

The previous reports have demonstrated that 3D echocardiography using reconstructed methods has overcome the limitations of 2D methods and provides an accurate measurement of LV mass.[58–60] However, there are still technical limitations in the clinical application of this method because multiple cross-sections should be acquired with or without ECG and respiratory gating. The real-time volumetric method, which requires only one cycle for 3D data acquisition, has overcome the problem of prolonged acquisition time. However, the image quality of first-generation RT3D echocardiography was comparatively poor because of relatively low spatial resolution. Thus, 3D echocardiography has not been widely used for the measurement of LV mass in clinical practice.

The introduction of the new-generation RT3D echocardiography has made both 3D data acquisition and 3D LV mass analysis an easy process, with good image quality using a standard ultrasound machine. This allows accurate and reproducible measurement of LV mass even in patients with LV hypertrophy.[52,61,62] In a recent report, more accurate estimations of LV mass were achieved with RT3D echocardiography than with 2D echocardiography.[62] In the study, it was possible to obtain adequate 3D data for LV mass analysis in 20 of 22 patients (feasibility 90%). The acquisition time of the 3D data by RT3D echocardiography was less than 10 seconds, shorter than the latest version cardiac MR data acquisition (10–15 minutes). LV mass is calculated by the average rotation method with eight apical cross-sectional images by manual tracing of the epi- and endocardial border of the left ventricle in each cross-sectional image at end-diastole (Figure 2.15). Finally, the entire LV myocardium is reconstructed (Figure 2.16), and the LV myocardial volume is calculated using the computer software. The LV mass can be obtained as the myocardial volume multiplied by the relative density of myocardium (1.05), please note 1.05, = relative density of myocardium. Regression analysis showed that LV mass determined by RT3D

A

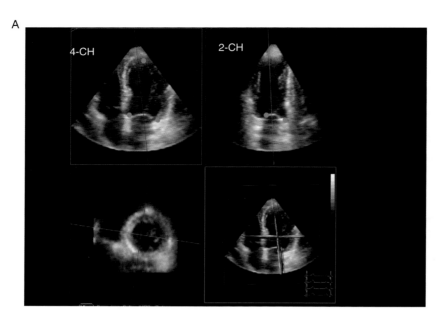

B

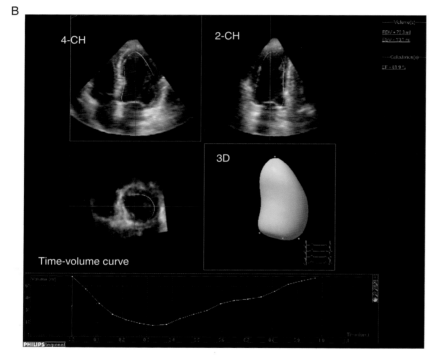

Figure 2.13 Semi-automated method for LV volume measurement in real-time echocardiography. (A) Anatomically correct apical 4- (4-CH) and 2-chamber (2-CH) views at end-diastole are extracted from the pyramidal dataset. Five anatomic landmarks are manually initialized: two points to identify the mitral valve annulus in the two apical views and one point for the apex. This procedure is performed in the frame at both end-diastole and end-systole. (B) Following manual identification of five points, the 3D endocardial surface is automatically identified (middle right). Finally, LV end-diastolic volume, end-systolic volume, and EF are automatically calculated, and a time–LV volume curve is shown (bottom).

echocardiography correlated well with LV mass determined by MRI ($r = 0.95$, $y = 28.9 + 0.851x$, = 20.3, Figure 2.17(A)), while LV mass determined by 2D echocardiography correlated less well with MRI-derived mass ($r = 0.70$, $y = 43.6 + 0.811x$, SEE = 58.0, Figure 2.17(B)). The correlation between 2D echocardiography and MRI for the LV mass measurement was less than that between 3D echocardiography and MRI. There were closer limits of agreement in 3D echocardiography for LV mass measurement than was demonstrated for 2D echocardiography. In addition, LV mass measurements by the new RT3D echocardiography system were highly reproducible.

Although breath-hold cine MRI has been used as a reference standard as it has been shown to be accurate and reproducible for determination of LV mass, cardiac MRI is costly, not widely available, not portable, and not suitable for patients with pacemakers or defibrillators, nor is it suitable for serial follow-up of patients. On the other hand, echocardiography is non-invasive, easy to apply, and has no risk of radiation and therefore can be used for serial examinations. Thus, monitoring of progression or regression of LV mass by RT3D echocardiography would be beneficial in the management of patients with LV hypertrophy.

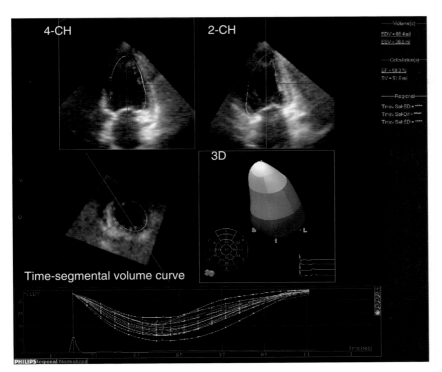

Figure 2.14 Time–segmental volume curve obtained from LV volume analysis in 3D echocardiography. Bottom curves show the time–volume curve in each LV segment divided as shown in the 3D image (middle, left panel).

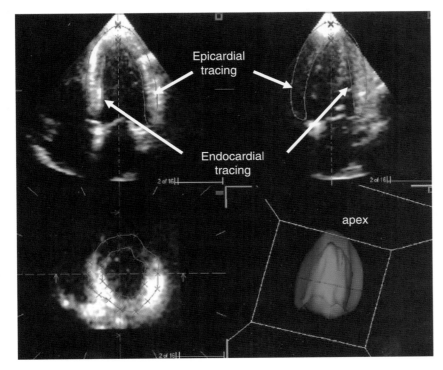

Figure 2.15 LV mass measurement by real-time 3D echocardiography. The epi- and endocardial border of the left ventricle is manually traced in each cross-sectional image at end-diastole. The entire LV myocardium is reconstructed (right lower image). The LV mass is calculated as the myocardial volume multiplied by the relative density of the myocardium.

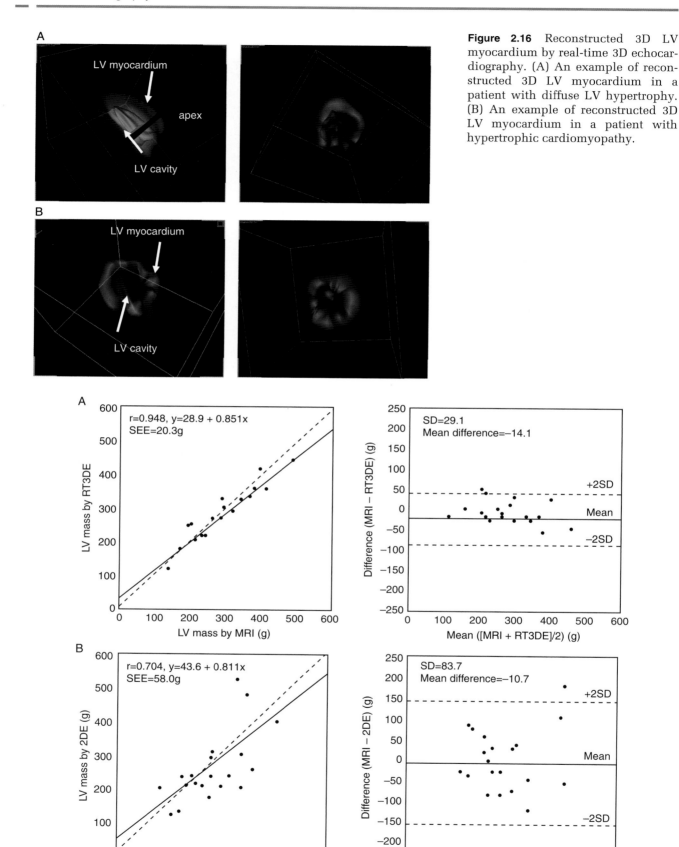

Figure 2.16 Reconstructed 3D LV myocardium by real-time 3D echocardiography. (A) An example of reconstructed 3D LV myocardium in a patient with diffuse LV hypertrophy. (B) An example of reconstructed 3D LV myocardium in a patient with hypertrophic cardiomyopathy.

Figure 2.17   (A) Regression analysis (left) and mean difference ± 2 SD between cardiac MR imaging and real-time 3D echocardiography (RT3DE) for LV mass. (B) Regression analysis and mean difference ± 2 SD between cardiac MR imaging and 2D echocardiography (2DE) for LV mass. Regression analysis shows that LV mass determined by RT3DE correlates well with LV mass determined by MRI, while LV mass determined by 2DE correlates less well with MRI-derived mass.

REFERENCES

1. Gottdiener JS, Bednarz J, Devereux R et al. American Society of Echocardiography recommendations for use of echocardiography in clinical trials. J Am Soc Echocardiogr 2004; 17: 1086–119.

2. Wyatt HL, Heng MK, Meerbaum S et al. Cross-sectional echocardiography, I: analysis of mathematic models for quantifying mass of the left ventricle in dogs. Circulation 1979; 60: 1104–13.

3. Reichek N, Helak J, Plappert T, Sutton MS, Weber KT. Anatomic validation of left ventricular mass estimates from clinical two-dimensional echocardiography: initial results. Circulation 1983; 67: 348–52.

4. Helak JW, Reichek N. Quantitation of human left ventricular mass and volume by two-dimensional echocardiography: in vitro anatomic validation. Circulation 1981; 63: 1398–407.

5. Schiller NB, Skioldebrand CG, Schiller EJ et al. Canine left ventricular mass estimation by two-dimensional echocardiography. Circulation 1983; 68: 210–16.

6. The Multicenter Postinfarction Research Group. Risk stratification and survival after myocardial infarction. N Engl J Med 1983; 309: 331–6.

7. White HD, Norris RM, Brown MA et al. Left ventricular end-systolic volume as the major determinant of survival after recovery from myocardial infarction. Circulation 1987; 76: 44–51.

8. Quinones MA, Waggoner AD, Reduto LA et al. A new, simplified and accurate method for determining ejection fraction with two-dimensional echocardiography. Circulation 1981; 64: 744–53.

9. Teichholz LE, Kreulen T, Herman MV, Gorlin R. Problems in echocardiographic volume determinations: echocardiographic–angiographic correlations in the presence of absence of asynergy. Am J Cardiol 1976; 37: 7–11.

10. Lang RM, Bierig M, Devereux RB et al. Recommendations for Chamber Quantification: A Report from the American Society of Echocardiography's Guidelines and Standards Committee and the Chamber Quantification Writing Group, Developed in Conjunction with the European Association of Echocardiography, a Branch of the European Society of Cardiology. J Am Society Echocardiography 2005; 18: 1440–63.

11. Erbel R, Schweizer P, Lambertz H et al. Echocardiography – a simultaneous analysis of two-dimensional echocardiography and cineventriculography. Circulation 1983; 67: 205–15.

12. Starling MR, Crawford MH, Sorensen SG et al. Comparative accuracy of apical biplane cross-sectional echocardiography and gated equilibrium radionuclide angiography for estimating left ventricular size and performance. Circulation 1981; 63: 1075–84.

13. Folland ED, Parisi AF, Moynihan PF et al. Assessment of left ventricular ejection fraction and volumes by real-time, two-dimensional echocardiography. A comparison of cineangiographic and radionuclide techniques. Circulation 1979; 60: 760–6.

14. Schnittger I, Fitzgerald PJ, Daughters GT et al. Limitations of comparing left ventricular volumes by two dimensional echocardiography, myocardial markers and cineangiography. Am J Cardiol 1982; 50: 512–19.

15. Koren MJ, Devereux RB, Casale PN, Savage DD, Laragh JH. Relation of left ventricular mass and geometry to morbidity and mortality in uncomplicated essential hypertension. Ann Intern Med 1991; 114: 345–52.

16. Ofili EO, Cohen JD, St Vrain JA et al. Effect of treatment of isolated systolic hypertension on left ventricular mass. JAMA 1998; 279: 778–80.

17. Liao Y, Cooper RS, McGee DL, Mensah GA, Ghali JK. The relative effects of left ventricular hypertrophy, coronary artery disease, and ventricular dysfunction on survival among black adults. JAMA 1995; 273: 1592–7.

18. Burke AP, Farb A, Liang Y, Smialek J, Virmani R. Effect of hypertension and cardiac hypertrophy on coronary artery morphology in sudden cardiac death. Circulation 1996; 94: 3138–45.

19. Bikkina M, Levy D, Evans JC et al. Left ventricular mass and risk of stroke in an elderly cohort. The Framingham heart study. JAMA 1994; 272: 33–6.

20. Ilercil A, O'Grady MJ, Roman MJ et al. Reference values for echocardiographic measurements in urban and rural populations of differing ethnicity: the strong heart study. J Am Soc Echocardiogr 2001; 14: 601–11.

21. Schiller NB, Shah PM, Crawford M et al. Recommendations for quantitation of the left ventricle by two-dimensional echocardiography: American Society of Echocardiography committee on standards, subcommittee on quantitation of two-dimensional echocardiograms. J Am Soc Echocardiogr 1989; 2: 358–67.

22. Collins HW, Kronenberg MW, Byard BF III. Reproducibility of left ventricular mass measurements by two-dimensional and M-mode echocardiography. J Am Coll Cardiol 1989; 14: 672–6.

23. Palmieri V, Dahlöf B, DeQuattro V et al. Reliability of echocardiographic assessment of left ventricular structure and function. J Am Coll Cardiol 1999; 34: 1625–32.

24. Park SH, Shub C, Nobrega TP, Bailey KR, Seward JB. Two-dimensional echocardiographic calculation of left ventricular mass as recommended by the American Society of Echocardiography: correlation with autopsy and M-mode echocardiography. J Am Soc Echocardiogr 1996; 9: 119–28.

25. King DL, Harrison MR, King DL Jr et al. Improved reproducibility of left atrial and left ventricular measurements by guided three-dimensional echocardiography. J Am Coll Cardiol 1992; 20: 1238–45.

26. Gopal AS, Keller AM, Rigling R, King DL Jr, King DL. Left ventricular volume and endocardial surface area by three-dimensional echocardiography: comparison with two-dimensional echocardiography and nuclear magnetic resonance imaging in normal subjects. J Am Coll Cardiol 1993; 22: 258–70.

27. Handschumacher MD, Lethor JP, Siu SC et al. A new integrated system for three-dimensional echocardiographic reconstruction: development and validation for ventricular volume with application in human subjects. J Am Coll Cardiol 1993; 21: 743–53.

28. Siu SC, Rivera JM, Guerrero JL et al. Three-dimensional echocardiography. In vivo validation for left ventricular volume and function. Circulation 1993; 88: 1715–23.

29. Handschumacher MD, Lethor JP, Siu SC et al. A new integrated system for three-dimensional echocardiographic reconstruction: development and validation for ventricular

volume with application in human subjects. J Am Coll Cardiol 1993; 21: 743–53.

30. Sapin PM, Schroder KM, Gopal AS et al. Comparison of two- and three-dimensional echocardiography with cineventriculography for measurement of left ventricular volume in patients. J Am Coll Cardiol 1994; 24: 1054–63.

31. Jiang L, Vazquez de Prada JA, Handschumacher MD et al. Quantitative three-dimensional reconstruction of aneurysmal left ventricles: in vitro and in vivo validation. Circulation 1995; 91: 222–30.

32. Gopal AS, Shen Z, Sapin PM et al. Assessment of cardiac function by three-dimensional echocardiography compared with conventional noninvasive methods. Circulation 1995; 92: 842–53.

33. Pandian NG, Roelandt J, Nanda NC et al. Dynamic 3-dimensional echocardiography – methods and clinical potential. Echocardiography 1994; 11: 237–59.

34. Roelandt JR, Ten Cate FJ, Vletter WB, Taams MA. Ultrasonic dynamic three-dimensional visualization of the heart with a multiplane transesophageal imaging transducer. J Am Soc Echocardiogr 1994; 7: 217–29.

35. Hozumi T, Yoshikawa J, Yoshida K et al. Three-dimensional echocardiographic measurement of left ventricular volumes and ejection fraction using a multiplane transesophageal probe in patients. Am J Cardiol 1996; 78: 1077–80.

36. Nosir YF, Fioretti PM, Vletter WB et al. Accurate measurement of left ventricular ejection fraction by three-dimensional echocardiography. A comparison with radionuclide angiography. Circulation 1996; 94: 460–6.

37. Buck T, Hunold P, Wentz KU et al. Tomographic three-dimensional echocardiographic determination of chamber size and systolic function in patients with left ventricular aneurysm: comparison to magnetic resonance imaging, cineventriculography, and two-dimensional echocardiography. Circulation 1997; 96: 4286–97.

38. von Ramm OT, Smith SW. Real time volumetric ultrasound imaging system. J Digit Imaging 1990; 3: 261–6.

39. Sheikh K, Smith SW, von Ramm O, Kisslo J. Real-time, three-dimensional echocardiography: feasibility and initial use. Echocardiography 1991; 8: 119–25.

40. Kisslo J, Firek B, Ota T et al. Real-time volumetric echocardiography: the technology and the possibilities. Echocardiography 2000; 17: 773–9.

41. Shiota T, Jones M, Chikada M et al. Real-time three-dimensional echocardiography for determining right ventricular stroke volume in an animal model of chronic right ventricular volume overload. Circulation 1998; 97: 1897–900.

42. Shiota T, McCarthy PM, White RD et al. Initial clinical experience of real-time three-dimensional echocardiography in patients with ischemic and idiopathic dilated cardiomyopathy. Am J Cardiol 1999; 84: 1068–73.

43. Schmidt MA, Ohazame CJ, Agyeman KO et al. Real-time three-dimensional echocardiography for measurement of left ventricular volume. Am J Cardiol 1999; 84: 1434–9.

44. Qin JX, Jones M, Shiota T et al. Validation of real-time three-dimensional echocardiography for quantifying left ventricular volumes in the presence of a left ventricular aneurysm: in vitro and in vivo studies. J Am Coll Cardiol 2000; 36: 900–7.

45. Takuma S, Ota T, Muro T et al. Assessment of left ventricular function by real-time 3-dimensional echocardiography compared with conventional noninvasive methods. J Am Soc Echocardiogr 2001; 14: 275–84.

46. Leotta D, Munt B, Legget M et al. Three-dimensional echocardiography by rapid free scanning from multiple transthoracic windows. J Am Coll Cardiol 1997; 29: 7055.

47. Mannaerts HF, Van Der Heide JA, Kamp O et al. Quantification of left ventricular volumes and ejection fraction using freehand transthoracic three-dimensional echocardiography: comparison with magnetic resonance imaging. J Am Soc Echocardiogr 2003; 16: 101–9.

48. Kawai J, Tanabe K, Morioka S, Shiotani H. Rapid freehand scanning three-dimensional echocardiography: accurate measurement of left ventricular volumes and ejection fraction compared with quantitative gated scintigraphy. J Am Soc Echocardiogr 2003; 16: 110–15.

49. Fukuda S, Hozumi T, Watanabe H et al. Freehand three-dimensional echocardiography with rotational scanning for measurements of left ventricular volume and ejection fraction in patients with coronary artery disease. Echocardiography 2005; 22: 11–119.

50. Sugeng L, Kirkpatrick J, Lang RM et al. Biplane stress echocardiography using a prototype matrix-array transducer. J Am Soc Echocardiogr 2003; 16: 937–41.

51. Kühl HP, Schreckenberg M, Rulands D et al. High-resolution transthoracic real-time three-dimensional echocardiography. J Am Coll Cardiol 2004; 43: 2083–90.

52. Arai K, Hozumi T, Matsumra Y et al. Accuracy of measurement of left ventricular volume and ejection fraction by new real-time three-dimensional echocardiography in patients with wall motion abnormalities secondary to myocardial infarction. Am J Cardiol 2004; 94: 552–8.

53. Gutiérrez-Chico JL, Zamorano JL, Pérez de Isla L et al. Comparison of left ventricular volumes and ejection fractions measured by three-dimensional echocardiography versus by two-dimensional echocardiography and cardiac magnetic resonance in patients with various cardiomyopathies. Am J Cardiol 2005; 95: 809–13.

54. Jacobs LD, Salgo IS, Goonewardena S et al. Rapid online quantification of left ventricular volume from real-time three-dimensional echocardiographic data. Eur Heart J 2006; 27: 460–8.

55. Sugeng Li, Mor-Avi V, Weinert L et al. Quantitative assessment of left ventricular size and function: side-by-side comparison of real-time three-dimensional echocardiography and computed tomography with magnetic resonance. Circulation 2006; 114: 654–61.

56. Gopal AS, Keller AM, Shen Z et al. Three-dimensional echocardiography: in vitro and in vivo validation of left ventricular mass and comparison with conventional echocardiographic methods. J Am Coll Cardiol 1994; 24: 504–13.

57. Gopal AS, Schnellbaecher MJ, Shen Z et al. Freehand three-dimensional echocardiography for measurement of left ventricular mass: in vivo anatomic validation using explanted human hearts. J Am Coll Cardiol 1997; 30: 802–10.

58. Kuhl HP, Franke A, Frielingsdorf J et al. Determination of left ventricular mass and circumferential wall thickness by three-dimensional reconstruction: in vitro validation of a new method that uses a multiplane transesophageal transducer. J Am Soc Echocardiogr 1997; 10: 107–19.

59. Gopal AS, Schnellbaecher MJ, Shen Z et al. Freehand three-dimensional echocardiography for determination of

left ventricular volume and mass in patients with abnormal ventricles: comparison with magnetic resonance imaging. J Am Soc Echocardiogr 1997; 10: 853–61.

60. Kuhl HP, Franke A, Merx M et al. Rapid quantification of left ventricular function and mass using transesophageal three-dimensional echocardiography: validation of a method that uses long-axis cutplanes. Eur J Echocardiogr 2000; 1: 213–21.

61. Mor-Avi V, Sugeng L, Weinert L et al. Fast measurement of left ventricular mass with real-time three-dimensional echocardiography: comparison with magnetic resonance imaging. Circulation 2004; 110: 1814–18.

62. Oe H, Hozumi T, Arai K et al. Comparison of accurate measurement of left ventricular mass in patients with hypertrophied hearts by real-time three-dimensional echocardiography versus magnetic resonance imaging. Am J Cardiol 2005; 95: 1263–7.

3 Coronary Artery Disease

Takeshi Hozumi and Junichi Yoshikawa

TWO-DIMENSIONAL ECHOCARDIOGRAPHY

Dobutamine stress echocardiography

Dobutamine stress echocardiography is useful for the diagnosis and prognostic stratification of patients with known or suspected coronary artery disease.[1-8] However, the conventional two-dimensional (2D) echocardiography technique has several important practical difficulties involved in the procedure. Multiple cross-sections of the left ventricle (LV) must be obtained from more than one window to visualize all segments of the LV and these must be obtained quickly and accurately to be comparable at each stage during the examination (Figure 3.1). In addition, operators must acquire the images of the entire LV quickly and accurately to be comparable between stages during 2D dobutamine stress echocardiography. Thus, even experienced examiners must take care to achieve accurate results from diagnostic dobutamine stress echocardiography[9] (Figure 3.2).

Segmental wall motion analysis

Two-dimensional echocardiography is a non-invasive, readily available technique for the evaluation of regional left ventricular (LV) wall motion. Semi-quantitative assessment of wall motion is applied in 16 segments (Figure 3.3), recently 17 segments. In clinical practice, visual assessment of endocardial excursion and wall thickening is most commonly used, although it is subjective and requires expertise.[10,11]

THREE-DIMENSIONAL ECHOCARDIOGRAPHY

Dobutamine stress echocardiography with previous 3D echocardiography

There has been no report applying reconstructed 3D echocardiography to stress echocardiography.

This technique may not be suitable for stress echocardiography because it requires acquisition of multiple 2D images at each stage. On the other hand, the real-time volumetric method, which requires only one cycle for 3D data acquisition, has overcome the problem of prolonged acquisition time.[12-19] In the dobutamine stress echocardiography study[19] using first-generation real-time 3D echocardiography, the 3D imaging allowed more rapid acquisition of the echocardiographic images than 2D imaging. In this 3D system, however, 3D datasets were sliced to view only the 2D images of the LV because this method could not visualize the 3D anatomic image immediately after scanning. In addition, the image quality of first-generation real-time 3D (RT3D) echocardiography was comparatively poor because of relatively low spatial resolution.[14,15] Consequently, 3D echocardiography has not been widely used for stress echocardiography in clinical practice.

Dobutamine stress echocardiography with new generation RT3D echocardiography

The recent introduction of a RT3D echocardiography system using a new matrix-array transducer has allowed the quick and simple acquisition of 3D datasets and 3D display of the entire LV with improved image quality using a standard ultrasound machine. Furthermore, RT3D echocardiography provides rapid display of multiple images in any number of different planes simply by rotating and cropping the acquired 3D datasets. A new generation of RT3D echocardiography provides an easy process for both 3D data acquisition and 3D analysis with good image quality using a standard ultrasound machine.[20-24]

Acquisition of 3D data

In dobutamine stress echocardiography with new RT3D echocardiography, images are acquired from

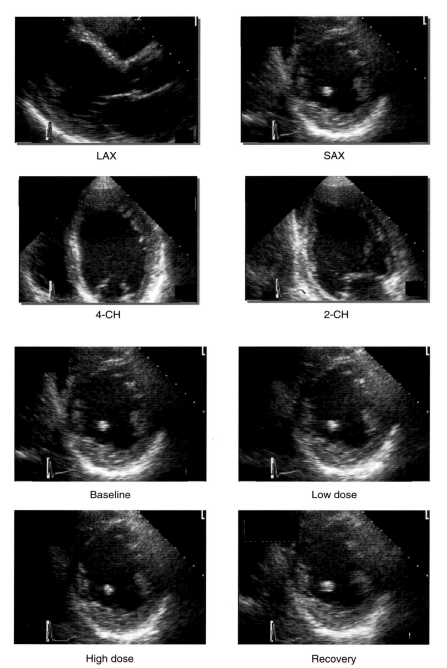

Figure 3.1 Parasternal long-axis (LAX) and short-axis (SAX) cross-sections, and apical 4-chamber (4-CH) and 2-chamber (2-CH) cross-sections must be obtained quickly and accurately to be comparable at each stage during dobutamine stress echocardiography. LAX = long-axis view, SAX = short-axis view, 4-CH = 4-Chamber view, 2-CH = 2-Chamber view.

Figure 3.2 Short-axis views at baseline, low-dose stage, high-dose stage, and recovery in dobutamine stress echocardiography.

the apical window. Two reference 2D images are displayed on the screen, helping the operator to position the region of interest with all targets being covered by the imaging volume. After visualization of the reference images, such as apical 4- and 2-chamber views, full volume datasets of the LV are acquired; four conical subvolumes of approximately 20° × 80° are scanned during 4 to 7 heart beats without moving the transducer (Figure 3.4). Electrocardiographic gating is necessary and, triggered by every other R-wave on the electrocardiogram, the four subvolumes are acquired. These four subvolumes are automatically integrated and entire pyramidal datasets of approximately 80° × 80° are obtained for the acquisition of the full LV volume.

Regional wall motion assessment
Regional wall motion of the LV can be evaluated using cropped planes. First, the acquired pyramidal volumes (anatomic image) are cropped from the apex to the base along the long axis of the LV, and short-axis views at various levels are produced (Figure 3.5(A)). Next, these volumes are cropped from the inferior wall and the apical 4-chamber image (long-axis cut plane) can be visualized as the reference. Then the apical 2-chamber image and the apical long-axis image are visualized with an inclination of the image plane of approximately 10–15° (Figure 3.5(B)). Thus, the various LV anatomic images can be obtained from the pyramidal volumetric datasets and, using these anatomic images,

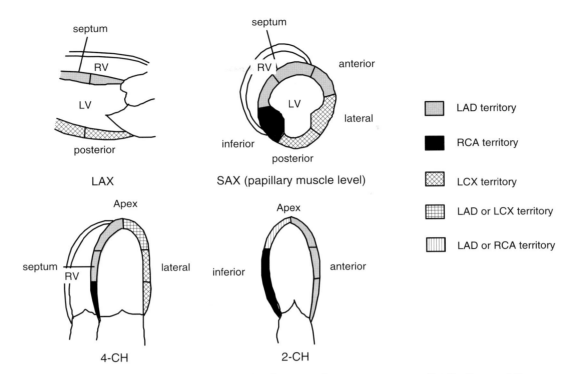

Figure 3.3 Schematic demonstration of the relationship between the coronary artery distribution and the corresponding left ventricular segments. LAX = long-axis view, SAX = short-axis view, 4-CH = 4-Chamber view, 2-CH = 2-Chamber view, RV = right ventricle, LV = left ventricle, LAD = left interior descending artery; RCA = right coronary artery; LCX = left circumflex artery.

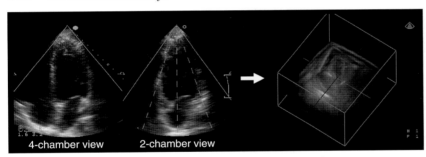

Figure 3.4 Acquisition of full LV data by new real-time 3D echocardiography. After visualizing the reference images (left), four conical subvolumes of approximately 20° × 80° are scanned without moving the transducer (middle). These four subvolumes are automatically integrated and the entire pyramidal (approximately 80° × 80°) dataset is obtained for acquisition of full-volume datadet (right).

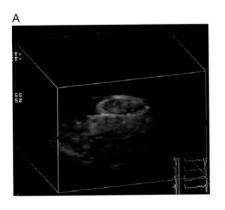

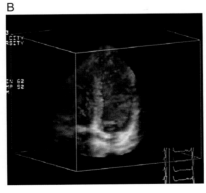

Figure 3.5 (A) The acquired pyramidal volumes were cropped from apex to base along the long axis of the LV, and short-axis views at various levels were produced. (B) These volumes were cropped from the inferior wall, and the apical 4-chamber image was visualized as the reference. Then the apical 2-chamber image and the apical long-axis image were visualized with an inclination of the image plane of approximately 10–15°.

regional wall motion of the LV is assessed by comparing baseline and peak stress images. An example of the detection of ischemia by RT3D dobutamine stress echocardiography is demonstrated in Figures 3.6–3.7.

Feasibility

A recent study[24] demonstrated that new RT3D dobutamine stress echocardiography enabled the acquisition of images of the entire LV from one echo-window without moving the transducer and allowed

End-diastole   End-systole

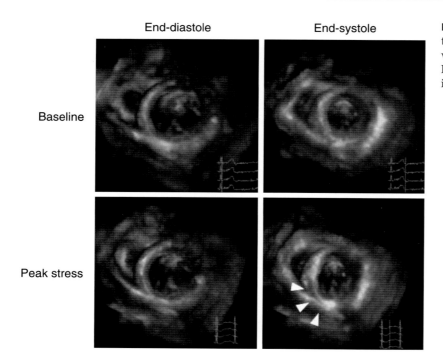

Baseline

Peak stress

Figure 3.6 Mid short-axis views by real-time 3D echocardiography in a patient with myocardial ischemia. At peak stress, LV wall motion abnormalities are shown in the inferior wall, as indicated by arrows.

End-diastole   End-systole

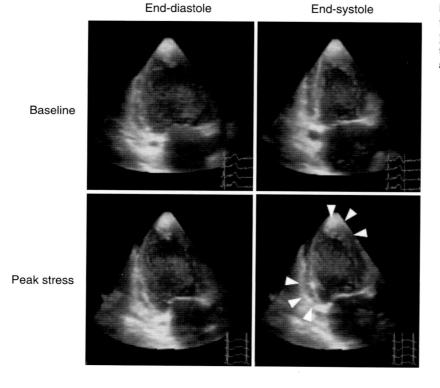

Baseline

Peak stress

Figure 3.7 Two-chamber views by real-time 3D echocardiography in the same patient as in Figure 3.6. Arrows point to the LV abnormality in the inferior wall and the apex at peak stress.

more rapid image acquisition compared to 2D dobutamine stress echocardiography. Additionally, the new RT3D dobutamine stress echocardiography provided an equally feasible and accurate assessment of myocardial ischemia as that provided by 2D dobutamine stress echocardiography. A comparison of the acquisition of adequate images between real-time 3D and 2D echocardiography was performed in each of four regions (apical, antero-septal, inferior, and postero-lateral) (Figure 3.8).

Real-time 3D echocardiography provided adequate images in 92% of all the regions at baseline, and 89% at peak stress. In comparison, 2D echocardiography provided adequate images in 94% of all the regions at baseline and 90% at peak stress. In each region, there were no significant differences in the success rate between real-time 3D and 2D echocardiography, both at baseline and at peak stress. However, the success rate of adequate image acquisition in the apical region tended to be higher by

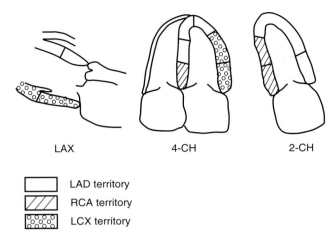

LAX   4-CH   2-CH

	LAD territory
	RCA territory
	LCX territory

Figure 3.8 Diagrams show the 16 regional wall segments and distribution of coronary perfusion. Left, long-axis view; middle, apical four-chamber view; right, apical two-chamber view. White area = LAD (left anterior descending), Slash area = RCA (right coronary artery), small circle areas = LCX (left circumflex artery).

RT3D than by 2D echocardiography, and the accuracy of diagnosing myocardial ischemia in the left anterior descending coronary artery territory tended to be higher by RT3D than by 2D stress echocardiography. These results suggest that RT3D echocardiography could accurately visualize planes for a precise comparison of the same segments in the apical region. Moreover, RT3D echocardiography allows analysis of the same segments in detail in different planes simply by cropping and rotating the 3D volumetric datasets. Thus, it is possible that myocardial ischemia can be detected in small regions by RT3D dobutamine stress echocardiography.

In the same study, the mean scanning time at peak stress, measured in 20 randomly selected patients, was 29 ± 4 seconds by RT3D echocardiography compared with a mean scanning time of 68 ± 6 seconds for a complete 2D echocardiographic acquisition. The mean scanning time at peak stress by RT3D echocardiography was significantly shorter than that by 2D echocardiography ($p < 0.0001$). These results suggested that RT3D echocardiography enabled us to perform dobutamine stress echocardiography more rapidly and simply than the conventional by 2D echocardiography.

Diagnosis of myocardial ischemia
The sensitivity, specificity, and accuracy of RT3D dobutamine stress echocardiography in the diagnosis of myocardial ischemia are 86%, 80%, and 82%, in comparison with myocardial perfusion imaging (SPECT), a gold standard in a recent report in 56 consecutive patients.[24] Those of 2D dobutamine stress echocardiography are 86%, 83%, and 84%, respectively. The sensitivity, specificity, and accuracy of these two methods were not

significantly different. Of the 168 major coronary territories in all the patients, myocardial ischemia was detected in 32 territories. 2D dobutamine stress echocardiography had a sensitivity of 75% and specificity of 89% for the detection of myocardial ischemia in each major coronary territory. In comparison, RT3D dobutamine stress echocardiography had a sensitivity of 75% and a specificity of 88%. There were no significant differences between RT3D and 2D dobutamine stress echocardiography in the accuracy of diagnosing myocardial ischemia in each major vascular territory (Table 3.1).

Limitations
New generation RT3D echocardiography needs four heart beats for the acquisition of the entire LV image data because the sector angle is only 20° × 80°, while first-generation RT3D echocardiography requires only one cardiac cycle for 3D data acquisition. However, the mean scanning time at peak stress within 30 seconds by RT3D echocardiography is better compared with a mean scanning time of more than 60 seconds for a complete multiple cross-sectional image acquisition in conventional 2D echocardiography. In addition, new generation RT3D echocardiography image quality has been improved compared to previous generation systems. We hope that future technical advances will allow real-time acquisition of a wider sector angle, while retaining image quality. Real-time 3D dobutamine stress echocardiography offers more rapid and simpler acquisition of the entire LV wall motion, and provides equally feasible and accurate assessment of myocardial ischemia, compared with 2D dobutamine stress echocardiography. The shorter study time and simpler technique should allow increased efficiency in performing dobutamine stress echocardiography studies. Real-time 3D echocardiography is expected to contribute to the widespread use of dobutamine stress echocardiography in the clinical setting.

Other methods using 3D echocardiography
Biplane and triplane display
Biplane (Figure 3.9) and triplane display (Figure 3.10) are another method for regional wall motion analysis in 3D stress echocardiography. This approach may be applied to exercise stress echocardiography. In the acquisition of 3D data in new RT3D echocardiography, breath holding for 5–10 seconds is required. In exercise stress echocardiography, it may be difficult to hold the breath immediately after exercise. In addition, breath holding may induce the reduction of heart rate due to an effect similar to the Valsalva maneuver. A study has shown that the use of biplane imaging during exercise stress testing reduces the

Table 3.1 Sensitivity and specificity of dobutamine stress echocardiography in the diagnosis of myocardial ischemia in the major vascular territories

	Sensitivity (%)			Specificity (%)		
	RT3D-DSE	2D-DSE	p	RT3D-DSE	2D-DSE	p
All territories (n = 168)	75 (24/32)	75 (24/32)		88 (119/136)	89 (121/136)	
LAD territory (n = 56)	80 (8/10)	70 (7/10)	1.000	93 (43/46)	93 (43/46)	1.000
RCA territory (n = 56)	79 (11/14)	79 (11/14)	1.000	93 (39/42)	90 (38/42)	1.000
LCX territory (n = 56)	63 (5/8)	75 (6/8)	1.000	77 (37/48)	83 (40/48)	0.508

DSE, dobutamine stress echocardiography; 2D, two-dimensional; RT3D, real-time three-dimensional; LAD, left anterior descending artery; RCA, right coronary artery; LCX, left circumflex artery.

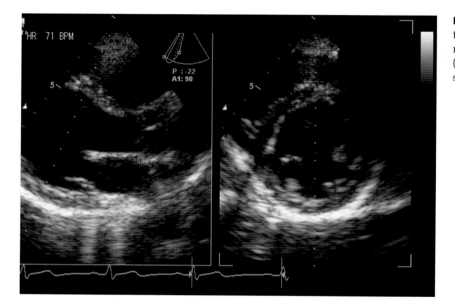

Figure 3.9 Biplane display in real-time 3D echocardiography. Without moving the transducer, both long-axis (left) and short-axis (right) cross-sections are displayed simultaneously.

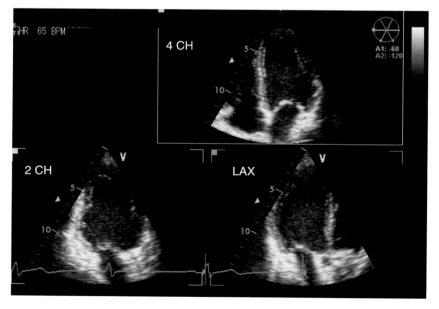

Figure 3.10 Triplane display in real-time 3D echocardiography. Without moving the transducer, four-chamber (upper), two-chamber (lower left), and long-axis (lower right) views are displayed simultaneously.

time required for data acquisition in healthy volunteers.[25] A 10 ± 7 second reduction in the acquisition time was reported for the biplane method compared to 2D echocardiography (28 ± 7 versus 38 ± 7 seconds). A reduction in acquisition time is a useful means to avoid decreasing the heart rate. Application of these displays to exercise stress echocardiography may be useful.

Nine short-axis views display

Nine consecutive short-axis cross-sections from base to apex can be simultaneously displayed from the 3D LV data in RT3D echocardiography. Using this display, wall motion in all the LV segments at peak stress can be compared with that at baseline in dobutamine stress echocardiography (Figure 3.11).

Assessment of segmental wall motion in 3D echocardiography

Recently developed semi-automated LV volume analysis software provides a quick calculation of 3D LV volume.[26] First, anatomically correct apical 2- and 4-chamber views at end-diastole are extracted from the pyramidal dataset on the first frame in the loop. Then, five anatomic landmarks are manually initialized: 2 points to identify the mitral valve annulus in the two apical views and one point for the apex. Then the same procedure is performed in the frame at end-systole. Following manual identification of these points, the program automatically identifies the 3D endocardial surface. Finally, the 3D endocardial surface during the entire cardiac cycle is demonstrated. Figure 3.12 shows an example of LV endocardial surface demonstrated by RT3D echocardiography in a patient with normal wall motion and ejection

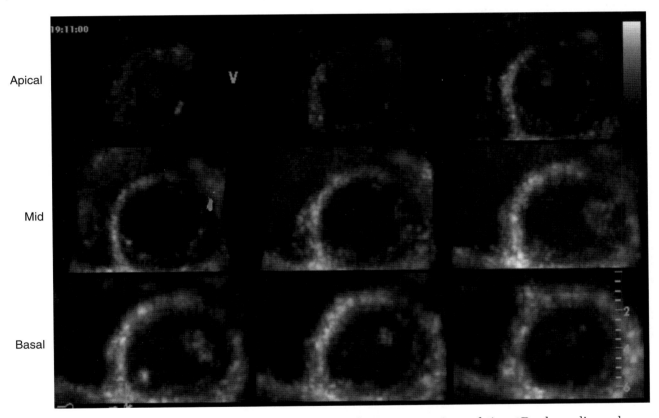

Figure 3.11 Display of nine consecutive short-axis views from base to apex using real-time 3D echocardiography.

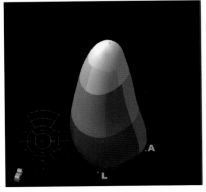
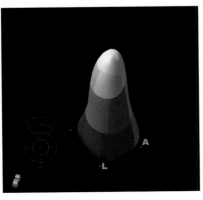

End-diastole   End-systole

Figure 3.12 An example of LV endocardial surface demonstrated by real-time 3D echocardiography in a patient with normal wall motion and ejection fraction (left: end-diastole, right: end-systole).

fraction. No apparent regional wall motion abnormality is shown. Figures 3.13 and 3.14 show similar displays in RT3D echocardiography in a patient with anterior myocardial infarction, and a patient with infero-posterior myocardial infarction, respectively. Wall motion abnormalities are demonstrated in the apical segments in Figure 3.13 and in the infero-posterior segments in Figure 3.14. Using this semi-automated system, LV end-diastolic volume, end-systolic volume, and ejection fraction can be automatically calculated. Not only entire LV volume but also segmental LV volume throughout one cardiac cycle can be demonstrated from the 3D dataset (Figure 3.15). These individual curves may be used for the quantitative assessment of segmental LV wall motion.[27]

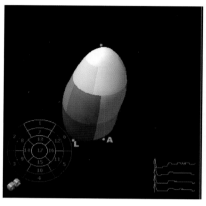
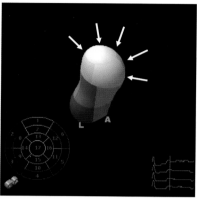

End-diastole

End-systole

Figure 3.13 An example of LV endocardial surface demonstrated by real-time 3D echocardiography in a patient with anterior myocardial infarction (left: end-diastole, right: end-systole).

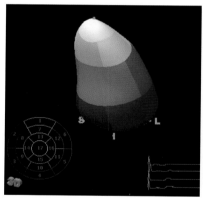
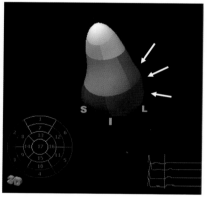

End-diastole

End-systole

Figure 3.14 An example of LV endocardial surface demonstrated by real-time 3D echocardiography in a patient with infero-posterior myocardial infarction (left: end-diastole, right: end-systole).

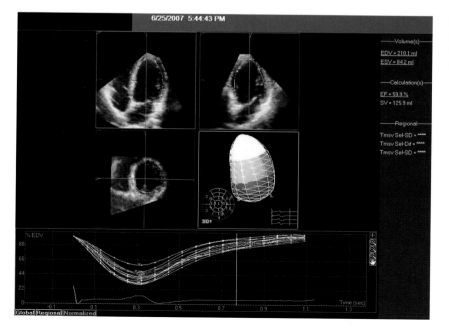

Figure 3.15 Segmental LV volume curves during one cardiac cycle obtained from real-time 3D echocardiography.

REFERENCES

1. Sawada SG, Segar DS, Ryan T et al. Echocardiographic detection of coronary artery disease during dobutamine infusion. Circulation 1991; 83: 1605–14.

2. Segar DS, Brown SE, Sawada SG, Ryan T, Feigenbaum H. Dobutamine stress echocardiography: correlation with coronary lesion severity as determined by quantitative angiography. J Am Coll Cardiol 1992; 19: 1197–202.

3. Mazeika PK, Nadazdin A, Oakley CM. Dobutamine stress echocardiography for detection and assessment of coronary artery disease. J Am Coll Cardiol 1992; 19: 1203–11.

4. Pellikka PA, Roger VL, Oh JK et al. Stress echocardiography. Part II. Dobutamine stress echocardiography: techniques, implementation, clinical applications, and correlations. Mayo Clin Proc 1995; 70: 16–27.

5. Geleijnse ML, Fioretti PM, Roelandt JR. Methodology, feasibility, safety and diagnostic accuracy of dobutamine stress echocardiography. J Am Coll Cardiol 1997; 30: 595–606.

6. Sicari R, Picano E, Landi P et al. Prognostic value of dobutamine–atropine stress echocardiography early after acute myocardial infarction. Echo Dobutamine International Cooperative (EDIC) Study. J Am Coll Cardiol 1997; 29: 254–60.

7. Chuah SC, Pellikka PA, Roger VL, McCully RB, Seward JB. Role of dobutamine stress echocardiography in predicting outcome in 860 patients with known or suspected coronary artery disease. Circulation 1998; 97: 1474–80.

8. Poldermans D, Fioretti PM, Boersma E et al. Long-term prognostic value of dobutamine–atropine stress echocardiography in 1737 patients with known or suspected coronary artery disease: a single-center experience. Circulation 1999; 99: 757–62.

9. Popp R, Agatston A, Armstrong W et al. Recommendations for training in performance and interpretation of stress echocardiography. Committee on Physician Training and Education of the American Society of Echocardiography. J Am Soc Echocardiogr 1998; 11: 95–6.

10. Hoffmann R, Lethen H, Marwick T et al. Analysis of interinstitutional observer agreement in interpretation of dobutamine stress echocardiograms. J Am Coll Cardiol 1996; 27: 330–6.

11. Picano E, Lattanzi F, Orlandini A, Marini C, L'abbate A. Stress echocardiography and the human factor: the importance of being expert. J Am Coll Cardiol 1991; 17: 666–9.

12. von Ramm OT, Smith SW. Real time volumetric ultrasound imaging system. J Digit Imaging 1990; 3: 261–6.

13. Sheikh K, Smith SW, von Ramm O, Kisslo J. Real-time, three-dimensional echocardiography: feasibility and initial use. Echocardiography 1991; 8: 119–25.

14. Kisslo J, Firek B, Ota T et al. Real-time volumetric echocardiography: the technology and the possibilities. Echocardiography 2000; 17: 773–9.

15. Shiota T, McCarthy PM, White RD et al. Initial clinical experience of real-time three-dimensional echocardiography in patients with ischemic and idiopathic dilated cardiomyopathy. Am J Cardiol 1999; 84: 1068–73.

16. Schmidt MA, Ohazama CJ, Agyeman HO et al. Real-time three-dimensional echocardiography for measurement of left ventricular volume. Am J Cardiol 1999; 84: 1434–9.

17. Qin JX, Jones M, Shiota T et al. Validation of real-time three-dimensional echocardiography for quantifying left ventricular volumes in the presence of a left ventricular aneurysm: in vitro and in vivo studies. J Am Coll Cardiol 2000; 36: 900–7.

18. Takuma S, Ota T, Muro T et al. Assessment of left ventricular function by real-time 3-dimensional echocardiography compared with conventional noninvasive methods. J Am Soc Echocardiogr 2001; 14: 275–84.

19. Ahmad M, Xie T, McCulloch M, Abreo G, Runge M. Real-time three-dimensional dobutamine stress echocardiography in assessment stress echocardiography in assessment of ischemia: comparison with two-dimensional dobutamine stress echocardiography. J Am Coll Cardiol 2001; 37: 1303–9.

20. Sugeng L, Kirkpatrick J, Lang RM et al. Biplane stress echocardiography using a prototype matrix-array transducer. J Am Soc Echocardiogr 2003; 16: 937–41.

21. Kühl HP, Schreckenberg M, Rulands D et al. High-resolution transthoracic real-time three-dimensional echocardiography. J Am Coll Cardiol 2004; 43: 2083–90.

22. Arai K, Hozumi T, Matsumura Y et al. Accuracy of measurement of left ventricular volume and ejection fraction by new real-time three-dimensional echocardiography in patients with wall motion abnormalities secondary to myocardial infarction. Am J Cardiol 2004; 94: 552–8.

23. Gutiérrez-Chico JL, Zamorano JL, Pérez de Isla L et al. Comparison of left ventricular volumes and ejection fractions measured by three-dimensional echocardiography versus by two-dimensional echocardiography and cardiac magnetic resonance in patients with various cardiomyopathies. Am J Cardiol 2005; 95: 809–13.

24. Matsumura Y, Hozumi T, Arai K et al. Assessment of myocardial ischemia using new real-time three-dimensional dobutamine stress echocardiography: comparison with exercise thallium-201 single-photon emission computed tomography. Eur Heart J 2005; 26: 1625.

25. Sugeng L, Kirkpatrick J, Lang RM et al. Biplane stress echocardiography using a prototype matrix-array transducer. J Am Soc Echocardiogr 2003; 16: 937–41.

26. Jacobs LD, Salgo IS, Goonewardena S et al. Rapid online quantification of left ventricular volume from real-time three-dimensional echocardiographic data. Eur Heart J 2006; 27: 460–8.

27. Corsi C, Lang RM, Veronesi F et al. Volumetric quantification of global and regional left ventricular function from real-time three-dimensional echocardiographic images. Circulation 2005; 112: 1161–70.

4 Right Ventricle

Florence Sheehan

Interest in the right ventricle (RV) has waxed and waned over the years. At one time it was even considered unnecessary for cardiac function because ablation of the free wall appeared to be well tolerated by experimental animals without reduction in cardiac output.[1] Interest in quantifying RV function surged briefly during the 1980s when thrombolytic therapy for treatment of acute myocardial infarction was under intense international study to prove that coronary reperfusion reduces mortality by salvaging ischemic myocardium. Attention turned away from the RV after recognition of its resilience to even prolonged coronary occlusion, even though RV function has a significant impact on prognosis independent of the left ventricle (LV).[2,3] Indeed more recent studies are demonstrating for a variety of cardiac conditions that the RV merits evaluation due to the impact of RV dysfunction on prognosis.[4,5] This chapter reviews the measurement of RV volume, function, and shape in the context of this chamber's anatomic structure.

ANATOMIC CONSIDERATIONS

The role of the RV is to maintain the forward flow of blood in the venous circulation. Because of the mechanical nature of this role, the function of both ventricles is inherently related to their structure. Operating at a lower pressure than the LV in the normal heart, the RV has a thinner wall and its contour is indented by the dominant LV. As a consequence RV shape is more difficult to describe in simple geometric terms than that of the LV.

Nearly all of our knowledge of ventricular fiber anatomy is for the LV. Through myocardial dissection studies, Streeter delineated the interweaving helical fiber pattern of the LV, which was likened to a wicker basket.[6] The fibers course in a continuum between the subendocardium and subepicardium. This helical pattern is key to LV ejection. Myocardial

fibers only shorten by 15%, so a normal ejection fraction cannot be achieved solely from narrowing of the ventricle by contraction of the more circular fibers. When the helical fiber layers contract, they contribute to LV stroke volume by shortening the ventricle.[7]

The RV also has a helical and continuous epicardial to endocardial fiber structure. Although the interventricular septum is generally considered part of the LV, the septum contains longitudinal fibers belonging to the RV (Figure 4.1). In contrast to the LV, which has superficial, middle, and deeper layers, the RV has only two layers in normal hearts, although a middle layer is seen in patients with unrepaired tetralogy of Fallot.[8] The middle layer contains circumferential fiber aggregates, referred to as 'constrictors', that act to reduce ventricular diameter,[9,10] and thus provide the 'triebwerkzeug' or driving force of the LV (see review of Krehl's

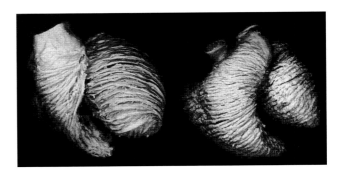

Figure 4.1 Stenocostal view of the middle layer in a normal (left) and malformed (right) heart. Note the lack of a middle layer in the normal right ventricle and the presence of a well-defined middle layer of fibers in the right ventricle of the malformed heart. (Reproduced with permission from Acta Anatomica, volume 138, Sanchez-Quintana D, Garcia-Martinez V and Hurle JM. Myocardial fiber architecture in the human heart, pages 352–8, copyright 1990, with permission from S Karger, AG, Basel, Switzerland.)

Triebwerk in reference 6). Without a middle layer the RV must rely more heavily on longitudinal shortening than does the LV.[8] Some investigators divide the RV chamber into two sections, the sinus and the conus. Fibers in the sinus free wall are mostly oriented obliquely with an average major radius of curvature of nearly 4 cm, whereas fibers in the outflow track are circumconal with a small radius of curvature of 0.8 cm.[11] The RV also undergoes torsion due to the contraction of its free wall fibers and not passively following the LV.[12] Contraction of the RV proceeds with a peristaltic pattern from sinus to infundibulum.[13] Dividing the RV into three anatomic components – inlet, apical trabecular, and outlet – facilitates analysis of congenital anomalies.[14]

The LV and RV are often analyzed as separate entities. However there are fibers that course between them at both superficial and deeper layers.[15] Therefore it is not surprising that the two ventricles interact functionally. In an electrically isolated free wall preparation, pacing of the RV resulted in little developed pressure in the LV, but pacing of the LV yielded near-normal RV pressure.[16] The authors wrote 'LV contraction was more important than RV free wall contraction for RV pressure development and volume outflow.' The interrelationship of LV and RV function has been demonstrated clinically: in patients with tetralogy of Fallot there was a significant correlation between LV ejection and RV ejection ($r = 0.67$, $n = 85$).[17]

Because the resistance of the pulmonary vascular bed is much lower than in the systemic circulation, the RV performs only a fraction of the external work compared to the LV. This can be seen from the shape of the pressure–volume curve, which is triangular for the RV, unlike the squared loop of the LV (Figure 4.2).[18] That is, RV ejection begins relatively early during the development of RV pressure, and continues even when pressure is declining. The advantage of this physiology is that the RV maintains its stroke volume with a lower energy expenditure, which can be estimated from the area of the pressure–volume curve. The disadvantage is that RV function is more sensitive to increases in afterload. This sensitivity is not an intrinsic property of RV myocardium, however, because the shape of the RV pressure–volume curve alters to resemble that of a normal LV under conditions of increased afterload such as pulmonary stenosis.[19]

LIMITATIONS OF 2D ECHO FOR MEASUREMENT OF RV VOLUME

The computation of LV volume from just two views, or even from a single view, is enabled by the regular shape of the LV, which lends itself to geometric modeling as an ellipsoid of revolution using the area–length method.[20] The RV on the other hand

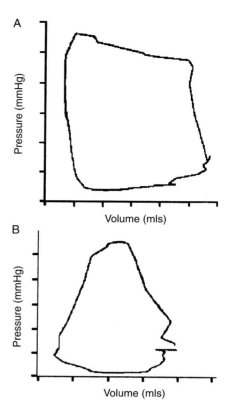

Figure 4.2 (A) Normal left ventricular pressure–volume loop. (B) Pressure–volume loop from the normal right ventricle. (Reprinted from Cardiology Clinics, volume 20, Redington AN. Right ventricular function, pages 341–9, copyright 2002, with permission from Elsevier.)

has such a complex shape that it has proven refractory to geometric modeling for volume estimation.

Several geometric models have been proposed and tested for the RV. The models can be grouped into three types, of which two were proposed initially for application to contrast ventriculograms acquired in the cardiac catheterization laboratory utilizing biplane views. The multiple slice method is not generally considered a geometric model, but when applied to biplane images it does make the assumption that the cross-sectional contour is elliptical[21,22] or hemi-elliptical.[23] The second type has the formula $V = kA_1A_2/L$, where A_1 and A_2 are the areas of the RV in the two views, L is the length of the RV long axis, and k is a constant. Depending on the value of k and how L is defined, the RV is compared to a parallelepiped, ellipsoid of revolution (area–length method), triangular prism, or pyramid.[24–26] When these methods were compared using in vitro hearts or models, the multiple slice method proved most accurate, although the area–length method also performed well, a surprise given the non-ellipsoid shape of the RV (Table 4.1).

In addition to the models developed for angiographic views are models that take advantage of ultrasound's tomographic rather than projection imaging. The formula $V = \frac{2}{3}AL$, where A is the area

Table 4.1 Accuracy of methods for measuring right ventricular volume

Modality	Publication (reference)	Reference method	n	Methods compared*	Most accurate: Criteria
Angiography	103	Cast	22	Multiple slice vs are length	Comparable: correlation coefficient, standard error, relative deviation
	104	Cast	40	Multiple slice vs area length	Comparable: correlation coefficient, percent error
	105	Cast	50	21 methods	Pyramidal: mean squared deviation, residual variance, correlation coefficient
	106	MRI	32	7 methods	Multiple slice and area length: mean squared difference
	107	Cast, model	27, 37	10 methods	Multiple slice: correlation coefficient, minimum absolute error, minimum signed error
2D Echo	29	MRI	33	5 methods	Biplane pyramid: $r \leq 0.86$ at end-diastole; $r \leq 0.82$ at end-systole
	33	MRI	10	5 methods	Crescent model: $r = 0.99$ at end-diastole, $r = 0.88$ at end-systole, r not significant for ejection fraction

*The number of methods includes variations such as number of slices or use of a regression.

in one view and L spans the RV in the other view, computes the volumes of numerous geometric figures that range from a prism to a crescent.[27,28] However the subcostal views that are required may be obtainable in only 52% of children older than 5 years.[29]

Even when an RV's shape fits a geometric formula, accuracy in RV or LV volume determination depends on the examiner's ability to locate image planes that yield the maximal area and long-axis length measurements. For instance, one study found that 95% of apical 2-chamber views were displaced anteriorly and superiorly to the apex, resulting in foreshortened views that underestimated LV volume.[30] Another study reported that even experienced examiners achieved optimal imaging, defined as ideal plane position ± 5 mm and ideal plane angle ± 15°, in only 32% and 48% of studies, respectively; none of the examinations was optimally positioned in all four standard views.[31] Use of a visual guidance system to assist in locating the apical 4-chamber view without foreshortening has improved accuracy in RV volume determination[32] (Figure 4.3).

These problems are magnified when dealing with conditions associated with considerable RV remodeling in response to the hemodynamic load,

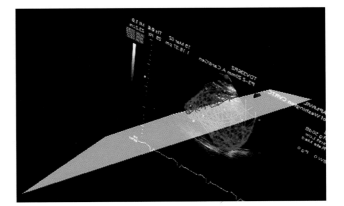

Figure 4.3 Visual guidance display to assist in acquiring images in anatomically correct standard views. Key anatomic landmarks are marked on initial 'scout' images for reconstruction of the RV using a catalog-based technique. The current image plane (translucent) can now be repositioned using the additional anatomic feedback. (Reprinted from the Journal of the American Society of Echocardiography, volume 16, Dorosz J, Bolson EL, Waiss MS, Sheehan FH. Three-dimensional visual guidance improves the accuracy of calculating right ventricular volume with two-dimensional echocardiography, pages 675–81, copyright 2003, with permission from The American Society of Echocardiography.)

such as pulmonary hypertension. Since RV shape can also change substantially in congenital heart disease, a given model may better fit diseased hearts than normal subjects, resulting in variable accuracy. Error in volume determination by both ellipsoidal approximation and multiple slice methods was significantly higher in normal subjects compared to patients with congenital heart disease,[29] probably because the RV had remodeled to a more ellipsoid shape in the latter. Reproducibility in volume determination is even more difficult to achieve because the lack of clear anatomic landmarks almost precludes locating the same anatomic image planes on serial studies.

In comparisons with magnetic resonance imaging (MRI) all two-dimensional (2D) echo methods performed poorly[29,33] (Table 4.1). For these reasons the 2D methods are not considered reliable for clinical use. Instead visual assessment is performed to gauge RV size relative to that of the LV. Normally the RV is only two-thirds the size of the LV in the apical 4-chamber view, the LV forms the apex of the heart, and the LV is round in short-axis views throughout the cardiac cycle. Deviations from this pattern may indicate RV dilatation, but careful examination of multiple views is recommended for confirmation of the diagnosis.[34]

THREE-DIMENSIONAL MEASUREMENT OF RV VOLUME

A major disadvantage of 2D methods for computing RV volume is their reliance on assumptions concerning the shape of the RV. These assumptions are embodied in the geometric figures to which the RV is compared. In contrast three-dimensional (3D) echo techniques eliminate these assumptions because the RV is reconstructed directly from image data.

MULTIPLE SLICE METHOD

The multiple slice method as applied to 3D data is independent of geometric assumptions. As a result even pathologically misshapen ventricles, as are commonly found in congenital heart defects, can be measured with satisfactory accuracy. The contours of the RV endocardium are delineated in parallel, evenly spaced planes, the area of each 'slice' is multiplied by the slice thickness (interplanar distance) to compute slice volume, and the volumes of the slices are summed to compute the volume of the RV. The method is referred to as trapezoidal integration when adjacent points on a slice are connected with a line, and as Simpson's rule when sets of three contiguous points are connected using a polynomial curve. For echocardiography the slices are of the short-axis view. For MRI some investigators advocate alternate slice prescriptions to more easily visualize

the tricuspid annulus and define the basal limits of the RV.[35]

The earliest publication on 3D echo for measurement of RV volume used the multiple slice method in conjunction with images acquired by the freehand scan technique and transducer tracking (Figure 4.4). The position and orientation of the 2D images was random rather than parallel.[36] The RV borders were traced in the images and then intersected with a stack of parallel planes spanning the distance from the apex to the base. The intersection of each plane with the traced borders produced a set of points that defined a contour for each slice from which RV volume could be computed.

In early attempts at volumetric imaging, multiple closely spaced images were acquired and interpolated to construct a solid volume of image data. The interpolated image volume was then sliced from apex to base into parallel short-axis tomograms from which the RV endocardial contour could be traced to compute volume. The spacing of the images was mechanically controlled to achieve rotational, fan-like, or parallel planes. Two studies performed on in vitro hearts reported good accuracy. Pini et al traced the RV borders in up to 49 parallel planes and found that the volumes of the summed slices

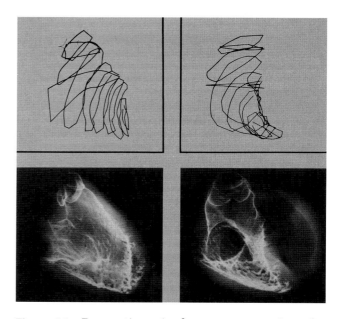

Figure 4.4 Perspective wire-frame representation of a 3D echocardiographic dataset (top) and double contrast radiographs (bottom) of the same calf heart. The left panels are in an orientation corresponding to a right anterior oblique projection, whereas the right panels are similar to a left anterior oblique projection. (Reprinted from the Journal of the American College of Cardiology, volume 8, Linker DT, Moritz WE, Pearlman AS. A new three-dimensional echocardiographic method of right ventricular volume measurement: in vitro validation, pages 101–6, copyright 1986, with permission from the American College of Cardiology Foundation.)

agreed well with MRI ($r = 0.97$, standard error of the estimate (SEE) 2.55 ml, $n = 14$ in vitro hearts).[37] Heusch et al also reported good accuracy for RV volume determination from images acquired at 1° angular rotational increments and traced from 2 mm slices ($r^2 = 0.93$, $n = 8$ in vitro porcine heart models).[38]

However the accuracy measured in vivo was less consistent. Papavassiliou et al reported better accuracy for RV volume than for function in children with congenital heart disease from rotations at 5 or 10° increments and tracings of 3 to 3.5 mm slices ($r = 0.95$ for end-diastolic and end-systolic volume, $r = 0.80$ for ejection fraction).[39] Vogel et al obtained good agreement between the volumes of the summed slices with MRI at end-diastole ($r = 0.95$) but not at end-systole ($r = 0.751$) in a population that included 11 pediatric patients with congenital heart disease even though they traced the RV borders every 2 mm; they also observed poor accuracy for measuring RV mass ($r = 0.65$).[40] Fujimoto et al obtained close agreement between 3D echo and MRI at both end-diastole ($r = 0.94$) and end-systole ($r = 0.97$) but not for ejection fraction ($r = 0.90$) in a population limited to normal subjects.[41] El Rahman et al examined 21 patients with repaired tetralogy of Fallot and obtained a similar agreement between 3D echo and MRI after tracing the RV borders from 1 mm slices ($r = 0.95$ at end-diastole, $r = 0.93$ at end-systole).[42] Thus despite time-consuming postprocessing, the assembly of densely spaced 2D images into 3D image volumes did not always provide adequate accuracy in RV volume determination for clinical application. Indeed, increasing slice thickness from 1 mm to 3.5 mm did not appear to affect the measurement accuracy.

The development of the matrix-array transducer has enabled the acquisition of the entire volume of image data at multiple time points through the cardiac cycle. An important advantage of this '3D/4D' echo is speed of image acquisition, which visualizes an entire segment of the heart in a single heart beat without need to average the data of multiple beats. In addition, 3D/4D echo reduces reliance on sonographer skill for measurement of LV volume,[43] although this has not been tested for the RV. A disadvantage is that the RV cannot be imaged in its entirety in a significant number of adult patients during the single apical scan that is most commonly employed to acquire the image data.

Testing of the first 3D/4D echo machine (Volumetrics Medical Imaging, Durham, NC) demonstrated excellent accuracy for RV volume in vitro.[44,45] However there was only fair agreement in RV stroke volume with measurements by flow probe in experimental animals ($r = 0.80$, $n = 6$ sheep studied at 14 hemodynamic conditions).[46] Another study in normal subjects reported no significant difference between 3D RV stroke volume and 2D LV stroke volume, but did not report the correlation.[45] In patients with pulmonary hypertension, correlation was poor between 3D echo and MRI for RV ejection fraction ($r = 0.60$; $n = 9$ patients).[47] However this early product had limited spatial resolution that may have made it difficult to analyze in vivo studies. Also the sector was too small for enlarged RVs.[47]

Currently available 3D/4D echo equipment, also known as 'real-time 3D echo' (RT3DE) has higher resolution and is marketed by multiple vendors (Figure 4.5). As with previous generations of 3D echo imaging equipment, excellent accuracy was obtained when testing in vitro models ($r = 0.97$ for volume and $r = 0.96$ for free wall mass, $n = 10$ porcine models).[48] In patients with arrhythmogenic RV dysplasia, the accuracy of RT3DE was poorer than reported for the first 3D/4D echo machine ($r = 0.50$ for end-diastolic volume, $r = 0.72$ for end-systolic volume, $r = 0.88$ for ejection fraction, $n = 43$ patients, relatives, or normal volunteers), but RV volume was measured from only two apical views rather than from multiple slices.[49] Software is commercially available for reconstructing the RV from three views (Figure 4.6).

SURFACE RECONSTRUCTION

In this approach to 3D echo the RV is imaged in multiple 2D views whose spatial location and orientation are tracked and recorded. The borders of the RV are then manually traced and used to reconstruct the surface of the RV endocardium in 3D.

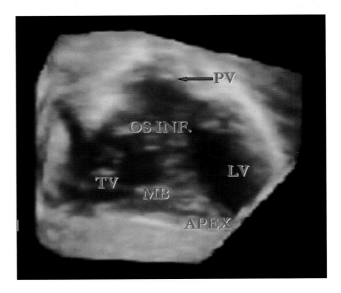

Figure 4.5 3D echo study of the RV from a matrix scanner. Subcostal 3D shows both inlet and outflow components of the RV. LV, left ventricle, MB, moderator band, OSINF, os infundibulum: opening of RV outflow tract, PV, pulmonary valve, TV, tricuspid valve. (Reproduced with permission from Dr David Sahn.)

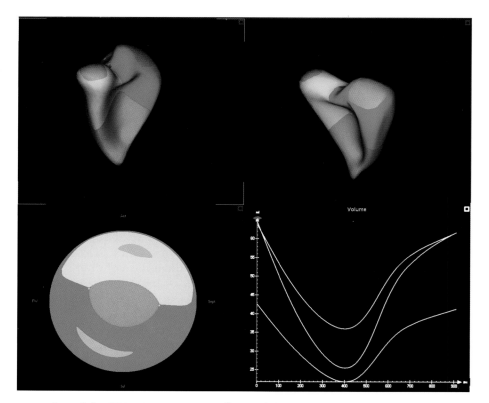

Figure 4.6   Reconstruction of the RV using commercially available analysis software. After the user traces three borders at end-diastole and at end-systole, the RV is automatically delineated in all remaining time points through the cardiac cycle. Coloring presents a model for assessing regional RV function. (Reproduced with permission from Tomtec Imaging Systems GmbH, Unterschleissheim, Germany.)

RV volume is then computed from the 3D surface. This approach permits image acquisition by freehand scanning, so that the image data can be acquired from whatever combination of acoustic windows and views provides optimal image quality in any given patient. As for volumetric 3D echo, manual border tracing is required from multiple image planes to obtain measurement of RV volume. The accuracy of freehand scanning for assessing the more symmetric LV has been widely validated. However few methods have been developed for the RV.

Surface reconstruction requires a method for recording the position and orientation of the 2D image planes in space, and software for creating the surface. Measuring the position and orientation of the transducer during cardiac studies has been performed using spark gap,[50] electromagnetic,[51] or mechanical positioning devices[52] (for a review, see reference 53). Nearly all tracking devices pose limitations: spark gap devices cannot be used to acquire both apical and parasternal views due to the need for clear line of sight between the transmitter and receiver, mechanical devices may hinder transducer manipulation optical devices are expensive and in-artial devices suffer from drift. In contrast the latest model of electromagnetic device (Ascension Technology, Burlington VT) has a flat transmitter that renders it immune to ferromagnetic interference from the hospital bed, so that it can be used in a normal clinical environment.

Given the complex shape of the RV, reconstruction of its endocardial surface requires more shape information than for the LV. This shape information is most commonly obtained by tracing RV borders in multiple views. A surfacing algorithm is then applied to fit a mesh to the traced borders.

Jiang et al reported on a method combining acoustic tracking and reconstruction from a spherical template[54] (Figure 4.7). They built in several technical features to improve accuracy, such as enabling review of the traced borders in a 3D window so that they could be checked against each other, e.g. to verify the intersection of borders traced from intersecting planes. Also, the surfacing algorithm accepted partial borders, so that data only needed to be entered where the endocardium was clearly visible. A disadvantage of the surfacing algorithm was its tendency to produce a sphere, thus rounding out a narrow apex or distal outflow track. The accuracy of their system was good on in vivo testing ($r = 0.99$ for end-diastolic volume, $r = 0.98$ for end-systolic volume, and $r = 0.98$ for ejection fraction, $n = 5$ dogs instrumented with intracavitary balloons and imaged under varying hemodynamic conditions). These investigators also obtained good accuracy for measuring RV free wall mass ($r = 0.985$, $n = 12$ dogs).[55]

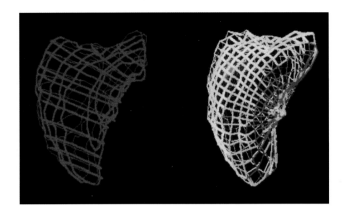

Figure 4.7 (A) Reconstructed traced borders of a beating RV, with inlet region at the upper left, apex below, and outlet at the upper right. Left Diastolic traces (in red) right systolic traces (in green) are shown combined with the corresponding surface used for volume calculation. (Reproduced with permission from Drs Leng Jiang and Robert E Levine.)

Buckey et al placed the transducer in a tilt-frame that measured its angle as it was swept from side to side in a fixed location in 5° increments. The image planes defined a series of wedges whose volumes were computed and summed to determine RV volume. Accuracy in vitro was good ($r = 0.95$, $r = 0.96$, respectively, $n = 20$ human heart models) for short-axis and apical scanning.[56] However it is necessary for the entire RV to be visualized from a single transducer position.

The piecewise smooth subdivision surface method was developed to avoid the limitations of earlier algorithms. Piecewise smooth subdivision surfaces[57–59] were used in the Pixar movies 'Toy Story II' and 'Monsters Inc'. In this method, a triangulated control mesh is designed as a model for each ventricle's endocardium and epicardium. The method allows parts of the control mesh to be marked as sharp, allowing for creases around valve orifices and along the RV free wall to septal edge in the final piecewise smooth subdivision surface (Figure 4.8). The control mesh is fit to the manually traced borders of the ventricle, valves, papillary muscles, apex, and other anatomic landmarks in a process that minimizes a penalized least-squares criterion that trades off fidelity to the borders against surface smoothness. The mitral and tricuspid annuli are fitted using a four-term Fourier series approximation.[60] Points traced from the aortic and pulmonic valves are fitted to a circle. Ventricular volume is computed by summing the signed volumes of the tetrahedra formed by connecting a point in space with the vertices of each triangular face on the reconstructed 3D surface. With the piecewise smooth subdivision method, the reconstruction avoids the rounding associated with some spherical templates. Instead this method incorporates knowledge about the

locations of sharp edges and of regions of complex shape requiring additional degrees of freedom to fit.[61] An advantage of the method is that the locations of anatomic landmarks identified on the images are conveyed to the reconstructed surface. These landmarks have aided in analyzing LV shape change from serial studies, although this has not been tested for the RV.[62] The landmarks also help to ensure that the same numbered triangles on the fitted mesh are assigned to corresponding anatomic locations from study to study and between hearts. To reconstruct the RV endocardium, the control mesh is fitted to 3D points sampled from the traced borders.[61] The piecewise smooth subdivision reconstruction method has been shown to accurately measure LV and RV volume and mass ($r = 0.99$ for RV volume, $r = 0.93$ for RV mass, $n = 10$ heart models). It is the only method shown to reproduce the 3D shape of the LV and RV with anatomic accuracy.[61,63] The method has been flexible enough to permit reconstruction not only of the RV and LV but also of papillary muscles, left and right atria, and liver.[64]

MAKING 3D ECHO FEASIBLE FOR CLINICAL APPLICATION

The 3D echo techniques described provide good accuracy for measuring RV volume, but require the tracing of the RV border in numerous images. To make these methods feasible for clinical application, several approaches have been tested to reduce the human workload. One approach is automating the image analysis. However despite decades of intense research effort, automated border detection of ultrasound images has been stymied by the inherently noisy nature of the images and the frequent signal dropout. For the RV this task is further complicated by the heavy trabeculation and prominent intraventricular structures as well as by the complex shape that has defied geometric simplification.

The remaining approach is to reduce the number of borders that need to be traced. For multiple slice analysis the practical question is, how few slices are needed? Chen et al performed an analysis comparing the true volume of experimental heart models with 3D echo volumes generated from varying numbers of slices. As would be expected, accuracy suffered as data input was reduced: $r = 0.97$, $r = 0.94$, $r = 0.78$, and $r = 0.75$ for 16-, 8-, 4-, and 2-slice analyses; similar results were obtained for measuring RV mass.[48] The authors concluded that the 8-slice model was the 'optimum choice for accurate and convenient measurement.' The method of Buckey et al required that 6–8 views needed to be analyzed.[56]

Munoz et al described a method that requires tracing the borders of only three mutually orthogonal planes and extrapolating the RV surface between these borders. However the requirement that the two longitudinal image planes contain the length of the long axis from the pulmonary valve to the RV apex is easily met only in in vitro hearts.[65]

Instead of making assumptions about RV shape, an alternative approach to reducing the workload of manual tracing is to make the reconstruction software more intelligent. A catalog-based method has been developed that utilizes knowledge of the expected shape of the LV or RV, and of the range of shapes that the ventricle can adopt in human dis-ease to reduce the required input data by 1–2 orders of magnitude compared to manually traced borders. The user acquires a 3D echo dataset and then traces 20–30 points – no whole or partial borders – from the images at key anatomic locations. The software relates the traced points by shape and anatomy to 3D reconstructions of the RV surface in a catalog containing normal and diseased hearts to recon-struct the new patient's RV (Figure 4.9). Volume measurement by catalog-based reconstruction req-uires about 3 minutes. On initial testing using a very small database of 3D reconstructions the mean

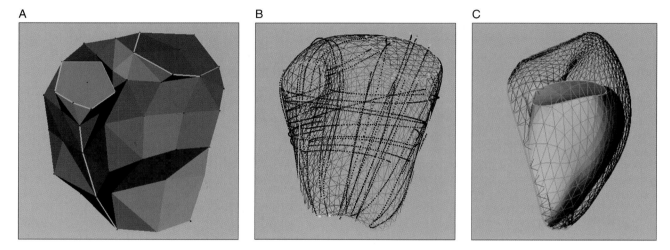

Figure 4.8   Reconstruction of the RV by the piecewise smooth subdivision surface method. Left, The triangulated con-trol mesh for the RV has edges marked as sharp to delineate the valve orifices and junction between the free wall and interventricular septum (green). Middle, Borders were traced of the free wall and septal walls of the RV, and of land-marks such as the tricuspid (cyan) and pulmonary (red) valves and apex (yellow). Final reconstruction (mesh) fits the control mesh to the traced borders, and then subdivides the triangles for smoothness. Right, Overlay of the RV recon-struction at end-diastole (mesh) on the end-systolic surface (solid) displays the descent of the base. This method was validated for accuracy in representing not only volume but also shape.[61,63]

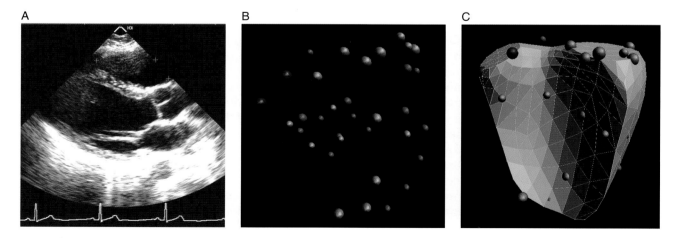

Figure 4.9   Knowledge-based reconstruction. Left, 2D echo image with traced right ventricular endocardium points (green crosses). Middle, Landmark points traced from multiple views, color-coded by anatomy. Right, 3D RV recon-struction generated from traced points with the aid of a database. This method has been validated for left and right ventricular volume determination.[66,67]

signed error was 7.3% of true RV volume as measured from 3D echo by multi-image border tracing.[32] A preliminary study of RV volumes in congenital heart disease reported good accuracy ($r = 0.98$, $n = 9$ patients with tetralogy of Fallot imaged by either 3D echo or MRI).[66] Accuracy for the LV performed using a more adequate database was good ($r^2 = 0.99$ for end-diastolic volume, end-systolic volume, mass, and ejection fraction).[67]

REGIONAL RV FUNCTION

Regional function assessment of the LV has a firm anatomic basis. The standardized 16 or 17 segment model into which the standard LV views are divided have correspondence to coronary artery territories.[68] However no equivalently standardized segmentation of the RV was presented in the recommendations for chamber quantification recently published by the American and European Societies of Echocardiography.[68] Since ischemia in the RV produces regional dysfunction out of proportion to the size of infarction, it is difficult to develop a segmentation plan based on ischemic dysfunction patterns for the RV comparable to that for the LV.[2] One scheme for semiquantitative assessment of RV regional function was to divide the free wall in the short-axis view into anterior, lateral, and inferior segments; global RV ejection fraction correlated well with the wall motion score index computed by averaging all of the segmental scores.[69] In the registry of arrhythmogenic RV dysplasia, wall motion was assessed in the same seven anatomically defined regions in echo as in angiography.[70]

There are few methods for quantitative RV wall motion analysis from 2D views because few of the geometric models developed for the LV can be applied to the RV. Radial coordinate systems do not fit long-axis views in general, and they also do not fit short-axis views of the RV due to the sharp angles at the junction of the septal and free walls. Rectangular coordinates do not fit crescentic contours well either. Because it does not rely on geometric assumptions about RV shape, the centerline method has been successfully applied for measuring regional RV contraction to angiograms, echo images, and MRI.[71–74]

Lacking consensus on standardized views of the RV, investigators have developed methods as needed for the question being addressed. The diversity of methodology is most prevalent in studies involving 3D analysis for conditions other than ischemic heart disease. In four studies of normal subjects, arrhythmogenic RV dysplasia, or congenital heart disease, the RV was divided into four circumferential regions, three vertical regions, or 9 to 12 regions created by subdividing short-axis slices.[74–77] One study carefully justified its segmentation

plan: McConnell et al observed a pattern of regional RV dysfunction in patients with acute pulmonary embolism by centerline analysis of RV wall motion. They also proposed diagnostic criteria for visual assessment of function in four regions of the RV free wall and then demonstrated the accuracy of these criteria.[78] It may be appropriate to use different segmentation plans for different disease entities. However it would be best if all investigators studying a given disease employed the same plan so that they could later compare their results.

Another approach to quantifying RV function is using surrogate parameters based upon a single view. The analysis is usually performed on the apical 4-chamber view, which is appropriate given the predominantly longitudinal contractile pattern of the RV.[79,80] The most common parameters are fractional area change and tricuspid annular descent.[81] Both of these parameters have been shown to predict outcome in heart failure patients.[3,82] A major disadvantage of the single view approach to RV function assessment is that errors occur when non-visualized regions fail to contract in a manner similar to that seen in the selected view. For example tricuspid annular descent deviated from its usually tight correlation with ejection fraction in a patient with apical dyskinesis.[83] Another study underscoring the importance of evaluating RV regional function throughout the ventricle reported that akinesia of the RV outflow track is associated with a poor prognosis in repaired tetralogy of Fallot.[17] Also tissue Doppler imaging revealed a relationship between regional dysfunction and abnormalities of electrical depolarization and repolarization.[84]

The little that is known concerning the 3D pattern of RV regional function comes from MRI tagging studies, which have documented the heterogeneity of normal RV wall motion,[85] confirmed greater long-axis than short-axis shortening,[79,80] quantified torsion,[12] and provided detailed analysis of the motion of the RV free wall toward the interventricular septum.[85]

RV SHAPE

Our understanding of ventricular remodeling derives from studies of the LV, which becomes more spherical when it dilates to compensate for volume loading.[86,87] This compensatory mechanism allows more even distribution of regional stress and improves ventricular efficiency. Measurement of the magnitude of these changes provides information on the mechanism, magnitude, and time course of remodeling and its effect on prognosis.

Study of RV remodeling has lagged behind that of the LV, because the RV's complex shape resisted simple geometric modeling. Also the early studies of RV shape were performed with the aim of measuring volume by angiography or 2D echo, not for analysis of remodeling.[88–90] Another problem is that RV shape can change substantially in congenital heart disease, so that a given model may better fit normal subjects than diseased hearts or vice versa,[91] resulting in variable accuracy.

In 3D imaging, the borders traced to compute RV volume using Simpson's approach define an RV surface whose base is truncated to exclude its two valve orifices. This simplified RV model has been applied in several studies of 3D shape. For example, remodeling in pulmonary hypertension was measured in terms of segmental volumes at five levels from apex to base.[92] Nielson et al used this approach in their elegant biventricular finite element model to investigate the relationship of RV shape to fiber orientation.[93] Young et al extended this method to describe the 3D geometry of the LV and RV in experimental mitral regurgitation in terms of distances, arc lengths, surface areas, and surface curvatures among regions defined by the nodes of the finite-element model.[94] Marcus et al reported that shape was less powerful than contraction pattern in predicting RV hypertension in neonates.[95] However their reconstruction method had not been validated for 3D shape analysis but rather for volume measurement.

Due to the difficulty in modeling the RV, research to analyze change in RV geometry in response to disease processes has been limited in scope. Studies of the impact of RV overload in congenital heart disease, pulmonary hypertension, and other conditions have concentrated on the shape of the LV and interventricular septum and its flattening or reverse curvature rather than on the RV (Figure 4.10).[96] At one time it was felt that regional RV wall stress analysis was impractical due to the RV's 'convoluted shape'.[97]

The RV contributes fibers to the interventricular septum. However several investigators studying RV shape have focused on just one wall of the RV instead of reconstructing the entire chamber. Sacks et al reconstructed the free wall of a normal canine RV in 3D from MRI data and characterized its regional curvature and the change in curvature through the cardiac cycle.[98] Moses and Axel reconstructed the septum and developed an analytic tool for quantifying the curvature of its RV surface throughout the cardiac cycle from MRI data.[99] Indeed virtually all ventricular shape studies in diseases involving the RV have focused on septal shape and its impact on LV rather than on RV function. For example, the degree of septal bulge into the LV cavity reflects the ratio of RV:LV pressure,[96] and depresses LV function in RV volume overload.[100] Compared to the LV, there are few studies of RV shape and remodeling.

Because an infinite number of shapes can hold the same volume, 3D shape should be analyzed from anatomically accurate reconstructions of the targeted chamber, such as those obtained using the piecewise smooth subdivision surface method. An additional advantage of this method is that anatomic landmarks identified on the images are conveyed to the final surface and can be utilized in computing parameters of geometry and shape. When the piecewise smooth subdivision surface method was applied to reconstruct the RVs of patients with pulmonary regurgitation following repair for tetralogy

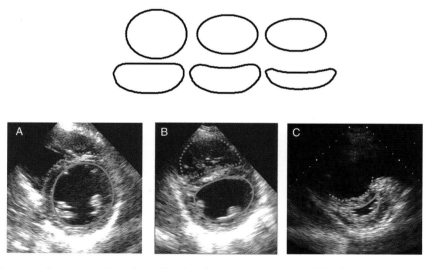

Figure 4.10 Top, Discrete shapes used to describe the shape sequence model. Shape factor is the pointer into this sequence and varies from a value of 1 for a perfect circle to 7 for an indented ellipse. (Reproduced from Azancot et al.[96]) Bottom, Short-axis echo views of a normal subject (A), a TOF patient with pulmonary regurgitation (B), and a pulmonary hypertension patient (C) illustrating the variation in the shape of the LV (solid green contour) and of the RV (dotted green contour) according to the level of hemodynamic load. (Reprinted from American Journal of Cardiology, Volume 56, Azancot A, Cowdell TP, Allen HD, Toscarll G, Debrux JL, Lamberti A, Sahn DJ, Goldberg SJ. Echocardiographic ventricular shape analysis in congenital heart disease with ventricular volume or pressure overload, pages 520–526. Copyright 1985, with permission from Elsevier.

of Fallot, two shape changes were seen: (1) bulging at the base lateral to the tricuspid annulus, and (2) tilting of the tricuspid annulus (Figure 4.11).[101,102] Similar shape changes were seen in pulmonary hypertension. These shape changes might have been difficult to recognize from short-axis images alone such as are prepared from volumetric 3D echo datasets, and probably would be excluded from analysis using RV models that truncate the base. Thus assessment of RV shape in volume and/or pressure overload conditions should not be limited to short-axis views. Rather RV shape should be assessed from 3D reconstructions generated from analysis of additional image plane orientations to obtain a comprehensive understanding of this chamber's remodeling pattern (Figure 4.12).

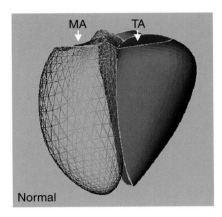
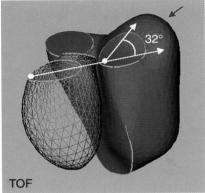

Figure 4.11 Reconstructions of the LV (green mesh) and RV (red surface) endocardium of a normal subject (left) and a patient with repaired tetralogy of Fallot (TOF, right). The TOF patient has severe RV dilatation due to pulmonary regurgitation and the LV looks diminished in comparison. The shape of the RV is characterized by widening at the apex (green arrow) and basal bulging (blue arrow) associated with tilting of the tricuspid annulus (TA) relative to the mitral annulus (MA) (white arrows). (Reproduced from Ventricular structure and function, Sheehan FH. In: The Practice of Clinical Echocardiography, Otto CM, ed, copyright 2007, with permission from Elsevier.)

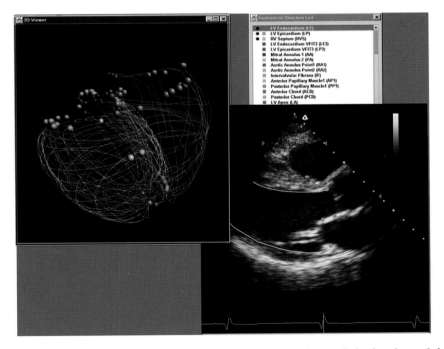

Figure 4.12 System for image analysis. The 2D images are reviewed (right) and the borders of the target organ and associated anatomic landmarks are traced. Using position and orientation information from the tracking system, the x, y coordinates of each border are transformed into x, y, z coordinates for display in a 3D window (left) where short-axis and long-axis and oblique image borders can be reviewed together. Here the red and green borders are traced from the left ventricular endocardium and epicardium, the blue and violet from the right ventricle, and the spheres from valve orifices, ventricular apices, and other anatomic landmarks. (Reproduced from Ventricular structure and function, Sheehan FH. In: The Practice of Clinical Echocardiography, Otto CM, ed, copyright 2007, with permission from Elsevier.)

REFERENCES

1. Sade RM, Castaneda AR. The dispensable right ventricle. Surgery 1975; 77(5): 624–31.

2. Laster SB, Ohnishi Y, Saffitz JE, Goldstein JA. Effects of reperfusion on ischemic right ventricular dysfunction. Circulation 1994; 90: 1398–409.

3. Zornoff LAM, Skali H, Pfeffer MA et al. Right ventricular dysfunction and risk of heart failure and mortality after myocardial infarction. J Am Coll Cardiol 2002; 39: 1450–5.

4. Bleasdale RA, Frenneaux MP. Prognostic importance of right ventricular dysfunction. Heart 2002; 88: 323–4.

5. Hesse B, Asher CR. Time to move to the right: the study of right ventricular performance: too long neglected. Clin Cardiol 2005; 28: 8–12.

6. Streeter DD Jr. Gross morphology and fiber geometry of the heart. In: Berne RM, Sperelakis N, Geiger S, eds. Handbook of Physiology. Section 2, Vol. 1. The Cardiovascular System (American Physiology Society). Baltimore: Williams and Wilkins, 1979: 61–112.

7. Sallin EA. Fiber orientation and ejection fraction in the human left ventricle. Biophys J 1969; 9: 954–64.

8. Sanchez-Quintana D, Anderson RH, Ho SY. Ventricular myoarchitecture in tetralogy of Fallot. Heart 1996; 76: 280–6.

9. Streeter DD Jr, Hanna WT. Engineering mechanics for successive states in canine left ventricular myocardium: II. Fiber angle and sarcomere length. Circ Res 1973; 33: 656–64.

10. Rushmer RF, Crystal DK, Wagner C. The functional anatomy of ventricular contraction. Circ Res 1953; 1: 162–70.

11. Armour JA, Randall WC. Structural basis for cardiac function. Am J Physiol 1970; 218: 1517–23.

12. Young AA, Fayad ZA, Axel L. Right ventricular midwall surface motion and deformation using magnetic resonance tagging. Am J Physiol 1996; 271: H2677–88.

13. Geva T, Powell AJ, Crawford EC, Chung T, Colan SD. Evaluation of regional differences in right ventricular systolic function by acoustic quantification echocardiography and cine magnetic resonance imaging. Circulation 1998; 98: 339–45.

14. Anderson RH, Ho SY. What is a ventricle? Ann Thorac Surg 1998; 66: 616–20.

15. Fox CC, Hutchins GM. The architecture of the human ventricular myocardium. Johns Hopkins Med J 1971; 130: 289–99.

16. Damiano RJ Jr, La Follette P Jr, Cox JL, Lowe JE, Santamore WP. Significant left ventricular contribution to right ventricular systolic function. Am J Physiol 1991; 261: H1514–24.

17. Davlouros PA, Kilner PJ, Hornung TS et al. Right ventricular function in adults with repaired tetralogy of Fallot assessed with cardiovascular magnetic resonance imaging: detrimental role of right ventricular outflow aneurysms or akinesia and adverse right-to-left ventricular interaction. J Am Coll Cardiol 2002; 40: 2044–52.

18. Redington AN, Gray HH, Hodson ME, Rigby ML, Oldershaw PJ. Characterisation of the normal right ventricular pressure–volume relation by biplane angiography and simultaneous micromanometer pressure measurements. Br Heart J 1988; 59: 23–30.

19. Redington AN. Right ventricular function. Cardiol Clin 2002; 20: 341–9.

20. Dodge HT, Sandler H, Ballew DW, Lord JD Jr. The use of biplane angiocardiography for the measurement of left ventricular volume in man. Am Heart J 1960; 60: 762–76.

21. Graham TP, Jarmakani JM, Atwood GF, Canent RV. Right ventricular volume determinations in children: normal values and observations with volume or pressure overload. Circulation 1973; 47: 144–53.

22. Gentzler RD, Briselli MF, Gault JH. Angiographic estimation of right ventricular volume in man. Circulation 1974; 50: 324–30.

23. Boak JG, Bove AA, Kreulen T, Spann JF. A geometric basis for calculation of right ventricular volume in man. Cathet Cardiovasc Diagn 1977; 3: 217–30.

24. Arcilla RA, Tsai P, Thilenius O, Ranniger K. Angiographic method for volume estimation of right and left ventricles. Chest 1971; 60: 446–54.

25. Fisher EA, DuBrow IW, Hastreiter AR. Right ventricular volume in congenital heart disease. Am J Cardiol 1975; 36: 67–75.

26. Ferlinz J, Gorlin R, Cohn PF, Herman MW. Right ventricular performance in patients with coronary artery disease. Circulation 1975; 52: 608–15.

27. Levine RA, Gibson TC, Aretz T et al. Echocardiographic measurement of right ventricular volume. Circulation 1984; 69: 497–505.

28. Denslow S. An ellipsoidal shell model for volume estimation of the right ventricle from magnetic resonance images. Acad Radiol 1994; 1: 345–51.

29. Helbing WA, Bosch HG, Maliepaard C et al. Comparison of echocardiographic methods with magnetic resonance imaging for assessment of right ventricular function in children. Am J Cardiol 1995; 76: 589–94.

30. Erbel R, Schweizer P, Lambertz H et al. Echoventriculography – a simultaneous analysis of two-dimensional echocardiography and cineventriculography. Circulation 1983; 67: 205–15.

31. King DL, Harrison MR, King DL Jr et al. Ultrasound beam orientation during standard two-dimensional imaging: assessment by three-dimensional echocardiography. J Am Soc Echocardiogr 1992; 5: 569–76.

32. Dorosz J, Bolson EL, Waiss MS, Sheehan FH. Three-dimensional visual guidance improves the accuracy of calculating right ventricular volume with two-dimensional echocardiography. J Am Soc Echocardiogr 2003; 16: 675–81.

33. Aebischer N, Meuli R, Jeanrenaud X, Koerfer J, Kappenberger L. An echocardiographic and magnetic resonance imaging comparative study of right ventricular volume determination. Int J Card Imag 1998; 14: 271–8.

34. Bleeker GB, Steendijk P, Holman ER et al. Assessing right ventricular function: the role of echocardiography and complementary technologies. Heart 2006; 92(Suppl I): i19–26.

35. Strugnell WE, Slaughter RE, Riley RA, Trotter AJ, Bartlett H. Modified RV short axis series – a new method for cardiac MRI measurement of right ventricular volumes. J Cardiovasc Magn Res 2005; 7: 769–74.

36. Linker D, Moritz W, Pearlman A. A new three-dimensional echocardiographic method of right ventricular volume measurement: in vitro validation. J Am Coll Cardiol 1986; 8: 101–6.

37. Pini R, Giannazzo G, Bari MD et al. Transthoracic three-dimensional echocardiographic reconstruction of left and right ventricles: in vitro validation and comparison with magnetic resonance imaging. Am Heart J 1997; 133: 221–9.

38. Heusch A, Koch JA, Krogmann ON, Korbmacher B, Bourgeois M. Volumetric analyses of the right and left ventricle in a porcine heart model: comparison of three-dimensional echocardiography, magnetic resonance imaging, and angiocardiography. Eur J Ultrasound 1999; 9: 245–55.

39. Papavassiliou DP, Parks WJ, Hopkins KL, Fyfe DA. Three-dimensional echocardiographic measurement of right ventricular volume in children with congenital heart disease validated by magnetic resonance imaging. J Am Soc Echocardiogr 1998; 11: 770–7.

40. Vogel M, Gutberlet M, Dittrich S, Hosten N, Lange PE. Comparison of transthoracic three dimensional echocardiography with magnetic resonance imaging in the assessment of right ventricular volume and mass. Heart 1997; 78: 127–30.

41. Fujimoto S, Mizuno R, Nakagawa Y, Dohi K, Nakano H. Estimation of the right ventricular volume and ejection fraction by transthoracic three-dimensional echocardiography. Int J Card Imag 1998; 14: 385–90.

42. El Rahman MYA, Abdul-Khaliq H, Vogel M et al. Relation between right ventricular enlargement, QRS duration, and right ventricular function in patients with tetralogy of Fallot and pulmonary regurgitation after surgical repair. Heart 2000; 84: 416–20.

43. Chuang ML, Parker RA, Riley MF et al. Three-dimensional echocardiography improves accuracy and compensates for sonographer inexperience in assessment of left ventricular ejection fraction. J Am Soc Echocardiogr 1999; 12: 290–9.

44. Schindera ST, Mehwald PS, Sahn DJ, Kececioglu D. Accuracy of real-time three-dimensional echocardiography for quantifying right ventricular volume: static and pulsatile flow studies in an anatomic in vitro model. J Ultrasound Med 2002; 21: 1069–75.

45. Ota T, Fleishman CE, Strub M et al. Real-time, three-dimensional echocardiography: feasibility of dynamic right ventricular volume measurement with saline contrast. Am Heart J 1999; 137: 958–66.

46. Shiota T, Jones M, Chikada M et al. Real-time three-dimensional echocardiography for determining right ventricular stroke volume in an animal model of chronic right ventricular volume overload. Circulation 1998; 97: 1897–900.

47. Angelini ED, Homma S, Pearson G, Holmes JW, Laine AF. Segmentation of real-time three-dimensional ultrasound for quantification of ventricular function: a clinical study on right and left ventricles. Ultrasound Med Biol 2005; 31: 1143–58.

48. Chen G, Sun K, Huang G. In vitro validation of right ventricular volume and mass measurement by real-time three-dimensional echocardiography. Echocardiography 2006; 23: 395–9.

49. Prakasa KR, Dalal D, Wang J et al. Feasibility and variability of three dimensional echocardiography in arrhythmogenic right ventricular dysplasia/cardiomyopathy. Am J Cardiol 2006; 97: 703–9.

50. Moritz WE, Pearlman AS, McCabe DH, Medema DK, Ainsworth ME, Boles MS. An ultrasonic technique for imaging the ventricle in three dimensions and calculating its volume. IEEE Trans Biomed Eng 1983; 30: 482–92.

51. Leotta DF, Detmer PR, Martin RW. Performance of a miniature magnetic position sensor for three-dimensional ultrasound imaging. Ultrasound Med Biol 1997; 23: 597–609.

52. Nikravesh P, Skorton D, Chandran K et al. Computerized three-dimensional finite element reconstruction of the left ventricle from cross-sectional echocardiograms. Ultrason Imag 1984; 6: 48–59.

53. Legget ME, Bashein G. Automatic border detection and three dimensional reconstruction with echocardiography. 1996; 12: 471–96.

54. Jiang L, Siu SC, Handschumacher MD et al. Three-dimensional echocardiography: in vivo validation for right ventricular volume and function. Circulation 1994; 89: 2342–50.

55. Jiang L, de Prada JAV, Handschumacher MD et al. Three-dimensional echocardiography: in vivo validation for right ventricular free wall mass as an index of hypertrophy. J Am Coll Cardiol 1994; 23: 1715–22.

56. Buckey JC, Beattie JM, Nixon JV, Gaffney FA, Blomqvist CG. Right and left ventricular volumes in vitro by a new nongeometric method. Am J Card Imag 1987; 1: 227–33.

57. Hoppe H, DeRose T, Duchamp T et al. Piecewise smooth surface reconstruction. Comp Graphics (SIGGRAPH '94 Proceedings) 1994; 295–302.

58. Hoppe H. Surface reconstruction from unorganized points. PhD thesis, Computer Science and Engineering, University of Washington, 1994.

59. Warren J, Weimer H. Subdivision Methods for Geometric Design. San Francisco, CA: Morgan Kaufmann, 2002.

60. Legget ME, Bashein G, McDonald JA et al. Three-dimensional measurement of the mitral annulus by multiplane transesophageal echocardiography: in vitro validation and in vivo demonstration. J Am Soc Echocardiogr 1998; 11: 188–200.

61. Legget ME, Leotta DF, Bolson EL et al. System for quantitative three dimensional echocardiography of the left ventricle based on a magnetic field position and orientation sensing system. IEEE Trans Biomed Eng 1998; 45: 494–504.

62. Hubka M, McDonald JA, Wong S, Bolson EL, Sheehan FH. Monitoring change in the three-dimensional shape of the human left ventricle. J Am Soc Echo 2004; 17: 404–10.

63. Hubka M, Bolson EL, McDonald JA. Three-dimensional echocardiographic measurement of left and right ventricular mass and volume: in vitro validation. Int J Card Imag 2002; 18: 111–18.

64. Hausken T, Leotta DF, Helton S et al. Estimation of the human liver volume and configuration using three-dimensional ultrasonography: effect of a high-caloric liquid meal. Ultrasound Med Biol 1998; 24: 1357–67.

65. Munoz R, Marcus E, Palacio G et al. Reconstruction of 3-dimensional right ventricular shape and volume from 3 orthogonal planes. J Am Soc Echocardiogr 2000; 13: 177–85.

66. Sheehan F, Ge S, Vick W. Monitoring right ventricular status in congenital heart disease (abstract). J Am Soc Echo 2005; 18: 559.

67. Wong SP, Johnson RK, Sheehan FH. Rapid and accurate left ventricular surface generation from three-dimensional echocardiography by a catalog-based method. Int J Card Imag 2003; 19: 9–17.

68. Lang RM, Bierig M, Devereux RB et al. Recommendations for chamber quantification: a report from the American Society of Echocardiography's Guidelines and Standards Committee and the Chamber Quantification Writing Group, developed in conjunction with the European Association of Echocardiography, a branch of the European Society of Echocardiography. J Am Soc Echocardiogr 2005; 18: 1440–63.

69. Lebeau R, Di Lorenzo M, Sauve C et al. Two-dimensional echocardiography estimation of right ventricular ejection fraction by wall motion score index. Can J Cardiol 2004; 20: 169–76.

70. Yoerger DM, Marcus F, Sherrill D et al. Echocardiographic findings in patients meeting Task Force criteria for arrhythmogenic right ventricular dysplasia. J Am Coll Cardiol 2005; 45: 860–5.

71. Sheehan FH, Mathey DG, Wygant J, Schofer J, Bolson EL. Measurement of regional right ventricular wall motion from biplane contrast angiograms using the centerline method. In: Computers in Cardiology. Long Beach, CA: IEEE Computer Society, 1985: 149–52.

72. Nakasato M, Akiba T, Sato S, Suzuki H, Hayasaka K. Right and left ventricular function assessed by regional wall motion analysis in patients with tetralogy of Fallot. Int J Cardiol 1997; 58: 127–34.

73. Yang P, Otto C, Sheehan F. The effect of normalization in reducing variability in regional wall thickening. J Am Soc Echocardiogr 1997; 10: 197–204.

74. Tulevski II, Zijta FM, Smeijers AS et al. Regional and global right ventricular dysfunction in asymptomatic or minimally symptomatic patients with congenitally corrected transposition. Cardiol Young 2004; 14: 168–74.

75. Menteer J, Weiinberg PM, Fogel MA. Quantifying regional right ventricular function in tetralogy of Fallot. J Cardiovasc Magn Res 2005; 7: 753–61.

76. Klein SS, Graham TPJ, Lorenz CH. Noninvasive delineation of normal right ventricular contractile motion with magnetic resonance imaging myocardial tagging. Ann Biomed Eng 1998; 26: 756–63.

77. Bomma C, Dal D, Tandri H et al. Regional differences in systolic and diastolic function in arrhythmogenic right ventricular dysplasia/cardiomyopathy using magnetic resonance imaging. Am J Cardiol 2005; 95: 1507–11.

78. McConnell MV, Solomon SD, Rayan ME et al. Regional right ventricular dysfunction detected by echocardiography in acute pulmonary embolism. Am J Cardiol 1996; 78: 469–73.

79. Fayad ZA, Ferrari VA, Kraitchman DL et al. Right ventricular regional function using MR tagging: normals versus chronic pulmonary hypertension. Magn Reson Med 1998; 39: 116–23.

80. Naito H, Arisawa J, Harada K, Yamagami H, Kozuka T, Tamura S. Assessment of right ventricular regional contraction and comparison with the left ventricle in normal humans: a cine magnetic resonance study with presaturation myocardial tagging. Br Heart J 1995; 74: 186–91.

81. Kaul S, Tei C, Hopkins J, Shah P. Assessment of right ventricular function using two-dimensional echocardiography. Am Heart J 1984; 107: 526–31.

82. Ghio S, Recusani F, Klersy C et al. Prognostic usefulness of the tricuspid annular plane systolic excursion in patients with congestive heart failure secondary to idiopathic or ischemic dilated cardiomyopathy. Am J Cardiol 2000; 85: 837–42.

83. Smith JL, Bolson EL, Wong SP, Hubka M, Sheehan FH. Three-dimensional assessment of two-dimensional technique for evaluation of right ventricular function by tricuspid annulus motion. Int J Card Imag 2003; 19: 189–97.

84. Vogel M, Sponring J, Cullen S, Deanfield JE, Redington AN. Regional wall motion and abnormalities of electric depolarization and repolarization in patients after surgical repair of tetralogy of Fallot. Circulation 2001; 103: 1669–73.

85. Haber I, Metaxas DN, Axel L. Three-dimensional motion reconstruction and analysis of the right ventricle using tagged MRI. Med Image Anal 2000; 4: 335–55.

86. Burton AC. The importance of the shape and size of the heart. Am Heart J 1957; 54: 801–10.

87. Dodge HT, Frimer M, Stewart DK. Functional evaluation of the hypertrophied heart in man. Circ Res 1974; 34–35(Suppl II): II-122–7.

88. Czegledy FP, Katz J. A new geometric description of the right ventricle. J Biomed Eng 1993; 15: 387–91.

89. Yim PJ, Ha B, Ferreiro JI et al. Diastolic shape of the right ventricle of the heart. Anat Rec 1998; 250: 316–24.

90. Matsumori M, Ito T, Toyono M, Harada K, Takada G. Influence of right ventricular volume and pressure overloads on assessment of left ventricular volume using two-dimensional echocardiography in infants and children with congenital heart diseases. Am J Cardiol 1997; 80: 965–8.

91. Helbing WA, Rebergen SA, Maliepaard C et al. Quantification of right ventricular function with magnetic resonance imaging in children with normal hearts and congenital heart disease. Am Heart J 1995; 130: 828–37.

92. Sukmawan R, Akasaka T, Watanabe N et al. Quantitative assessment of right ventricular geometric remodeling in pulmonary hypertension secondary to left-sided heart disease using real-time three-dimensional echocardiography. Am J Cardiol 2004; 94: 1096–9.

93. Nielsen PMF, Le Grice IJ, Smaill BH, Hunter PJ. Mathematical model of geometry and fibrous structure of the heart. Am J Physiol 1991; 260(Heart Circ Physiol 29): H1365–78.

94. Young AA, Orr R, Smaill BH, Dell'Italia LJ. Three-dimensional changes in left and right ventricular geometry in chronic mitral regurgitation. Am J Physiol 1996; 271: H2689–700.

95. Marcus EN, Munoz RA, Margossian R, Colan SD, Wessel DL. Echocardiographic assessment of the right ventricular response to hypertension in neonates on the basis of average-shaped contraction models. J Am Soc Echocardiogr 2002; 15: 1145–53.

96. Azancot A, Caudell TP, Allen HD et al. Echocardiographic ventricular shape analysis in congenital heart disease with right ventricular volume or pressure overload. Am J Cardiol 1985; 56: 520–6.

97. Leman RB, Spinale FG, Dorn GWI et al. Supernormal ejection performance is isolated to the ipsilateral

congenitally pressure-overloaded ventricle. J Am Coll Cardiol 1989; 13: 1314–19.

98. Sacks MS, Chuong CJ, Templeton GH, Peshock R. In vivo 3-D reconstruction and geometric characterization of the right ventricular free wall. Ann Biomed Eng 1993; 21: 263–75.

99. Moses DA, Axel L. Quantification of the curvature and shape of the interventricular septum. Magn Reson Med 2004; 52: 154–63.

100. Louie EK, Lin SS, Reynertson SI et al. Pressure and volume loading of the right ventricle have opposite effects on left ventricular ejection fraction. Circulation 1995; 92: 819–24.

101. Urnes K, Sheehan FH. Three-dimensional remodeling of the right ventricle varies under different loading conditions (abstract). J Am Soc Echo 2005; 18: 564.

102. Sheehan FH, Ge S, Vick GW III. The right ventricle in tetralogy of Fallot remodels to a different 3D shape from dilated cardiomyopathy (abstract). J Am Soc Echo 2005; 18: 515.

103. Lange PE, Onnasch D, Farr FL, Heintzen PH. Angiocardiographic right ventricular volume determination. Accuracy, as determined from human casts, and clinical application. Eur J Cardiol 1978; 8: 477–501.

104. Shimazaki Y, Kawashima Y, Mori T, Beppu S, Yokota K. Angiographic volume estimation of right ventricle: re-evaluation of the previous methods. Chest 1980; 77: 390–5.

105. Dubel HP, Romaniuk P, Tschapek A. Investigation of human right ventricular cast specimens. Cardiovasc Interven Radiol 1982; 5: 296–303.

106. Ernst W, Peter E, Juergen H et al. Evaluation of new software for angiographic determination of right ventricular volumes. Int J Cardiovasc Imag 2005; 21: 575–85.

107. Sheehan FH, Bolson EL. Measurement of right ventricular volume from contrast ventriculograms: in vitro validation by cast and 3 dimensional echo. Cathet Cardiovasc Interven 2004; 62: 46–51.

5 Left Atrium

Fabrice Bauer, Erwan Donal and Takahiro Shiota

INTRODUCTION

Anatomically, the left atrium is located on the rear side of the heart. It receives and expels oxygenated blood from pulmonary veins to the left ventricle during each cardiac cycle. The left atrium behaves as a conduit during early diastole, as a pump during late diastole, and as a reservoir while the left ventricle contracts.

The left atrial function has been identified as independent, pressure- and volume-related, and also linked to the left ventricular mechanic along with heart interaction in the chest.[1] Left atrial function is even more complex if we consider the body structurally and physiologically different to the appendage.[2]

Evaluation of left atrium function is routinely done in the echo lab by simply measuring M-mode diameter from the parastemal view or two-dimensional (2D) area from the apical view. Pulmonary venous flow velocities along with mitral inflow velocities interrogation give information on left atrial preload and afterload. Recent papers have pointed out the advantages of evaluating regional left atrial function by tissue Doppler imaging.[3]

Among the new technologies, three-dimensional (3D) echocardiography is complementary to conventional echocardiography, offering many other functionalities arising from full-volume visualization, navigation, and reconstruction. Three-dimensional echocardiography is naturally the direction any echo-cardiologist and sonographer should head for the next 20 years.

ANATOMY OF THE LEFT ATRIUM

The left atrium is divided into a posterior and an anterior half. The posterior half receives blood from the *four pulmonary veins*. In the upper posterior part enter the two superior pulmonary veins, whereas the two inferior pulmonary veins open into the lower posterior left atrium. The anterior portion called the *body* is continuous with the *left atrial appendage* (LAA). The left atrial appendage is a blind-ending saccule that projects anteriorly and then to the right over the external surface of the pulmonary trunk. Its inner surface is covered by musculi pectinati. From the atrium, the blood is emptied into the left ventricle through the mitral valve. The interatrial septum lies in front of the left atrium as well as to its right. The interatrial septum forms part of the anterior wall of the left atrium. The wall of the interatrial septum is smooth and has a small depression called the fossa ovalis. This fossa marks the location of the foramen ovale, a temporary aperture through which blood flows from the right to the left atrium before birth. Similar to the right atrium, there is a thin area located on the septum called the valvule of the foramen ovale.

Clinical 2D echocardiography

In routine echocardiography, it may be possible to image the left atrium from the left parasternal, apical, and subcostal window angles (Figure 5.1). A number of windows onto the left atrium are necessary for two principal reasons:

(1) A single transducer position is inadequate to see all the left atrial structures. For instance, the subcostal window gives only focused information of the interatrial septum. The left parasternal view provides inadequate functional imaging and truncated anatomy of the left atrium (the left atrial roof and the pulmonary veins outlets are often indistinguishable).[4] Finally, the apical view seems the most appropriate to obtain a full anatomic description and accurate functional assessment of the left atrium.

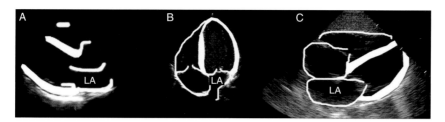

Figure 5.1 The three relevant views of the left atrium: the parasternal (A), the apical 4 chambers (B), and the subcostal window (C). Among these views, the apical imaging gives both dimension and functional information of the left atrium, thus should be widely employed.

(2) Routine echocardiography is a real-time 2D but single plane visualization of heart structures. A single window might be inadequate to see a localized abnormality requiring trivial tilting, displacement or probe rotation.

Three-dimensional view of normal left atrial components

When the left atrium is being imaged, the patient is instructed not to move during imaging and to breathe normally in the left lateral decubitus position as with other 3D ultrasound studies. Although 3D echocardiography allows acquisition of complete datasets that could be rotated in infinite cross-sections and eventually reconstructed for 'en face views', two scans are usually required to image the left atrium, giving the best spatial resolution of the investigated structure. The first scan starts with the parasternal view showing simultaneously two orthogonal planes, i.e. a long- and a short-axis view (Figure 5.2). An additional plane could be displayed with 60° angulation. The second scan is performed as illustrated in Figure 5.3 at the apical window depicting in real time two orthogonal planes or three with a 60° increment (Figure 5.4). The third subcostal scan is optional, and can supplement any view requiring additional coverage. From these views, it is easy to measure LA volumes and function, to slice the appendage, to navigate across the pulmonary veins, and to get on-line volume rendering of the interatrial septum and mitral valve.

Imaging the interatrial septum

The subcostal examination provides the best 3D image of the interatrial septum because the ultrasound beams are perpendicular to the septum. This window is ideal but does not preclude dropout from the fosse ovale that accounts for false positives. Therefore care must be taken to conclude in a communication between both atria or when calibrating the hole for atrial septal defect closure (Figure 5.5). Dropouts are more likely to be seen when scanning the septum from different locations. This holds true in children, but in adults this view is particularly disappointing and the parasternal should be preferred (Figure 5.2).

Imaging the left atrial appendage (LAA)

The LAA is a small structure suspended on the left side of the atrial body. Anatomically and mechanically different from the rest of the LA body, LAA dimensions and function are often evaluated by 2D transesophageal echocardiography (TEE).

In 2002, Valocik et al first calculated LAA ejection fraction by TEE 3D echocardiography from optimal cut-plane angulation of the LAA view at 135° with an interobserver variability markedly lower than for 2D echocardiography.[5] Subsequently, they found a significant linear relationship between LAA ejection fraction and Doppler late peak emptying velocity, one of the usual parameters of LAA function and thrombosis. More recently, Agoston et al imaged the LAA by transthoracic live 3D echocardiography from an apical approach.[6] They concluded that LAA scanning by this method was feasible, offering an improvement in LAA visualization by over 50% when compared to 2D echocardiography. Furthermore, patients with LAA thrombi on TEE had thrombi detected by live 3D echocardiography as well. This was also reported by Khan et al.[7] Figures 5.6 and 5.7 show two examples of the LAA from an apical and parasternal view, respectively.

Imaging the pulmonary veins

The pulmonary veins can be visualized from one single position. The apical window gives the most appropriate view, but the spatial resolution in the far field is problematic. In an optimal setting and an excellent acoustic window it should be possible to see at least three out of the four pulmonary veins, but in our experience it is difficult to incorporate more than two veins in a volume-rendered reconstruction (Figure 5.8). This may explain the limited number of publications on the pulmonary veins despite great interest in the field of supraventricular arrhythmia.

MEASURING LEFT ATRIAL VOLUME AND FUNCTION BY 3D ECHOCARDIOGRAPHY

Rationale for left atrial volume measurement

Left atrial volume and function measurements provide information regarding the prognosis and management of a large proportion of patients suffering

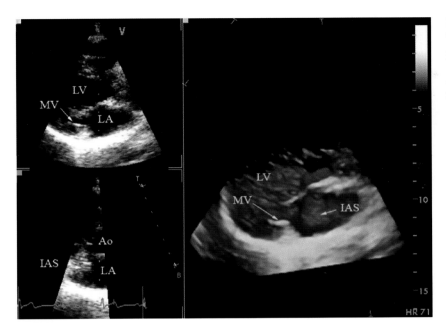

Figure 5.2 Parasternal view obtained with one patient. Top left shows a short-axis view while, simultaneously, bottom left shows a long-axis view and right displays a volume-rendered reconstruction. LA, left atrium; LV, left ventricle; MV, mitral valve; Ao, aorta; IAS, interatrial septum.

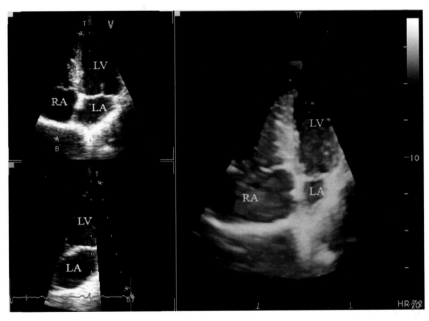

Figure 5.3 Apical view obtained with one patient. Top left shows a 4-chamber view while, simultaneously, bottom left shows 2-chamber view and right depicts a volume-rendered reconstruction. LA, left atrium; LV, left ventricle; RA, right atrium.

from cardiovascular diseases.[8] Echocardiographic M-mode diameter and 2D planimetry were the most frequently used diagnostic tool for characterizing LA dilation. From these two measurements, multiple equations were identified that correlate well with real LA volume.[9] However, these calculations are limited because they rely on certain geometric assumptions to calculate LA volumes which may introduce serious errors. In the evolving course of heart disease, the left atrium stretches more anterior-posteriorly than sagitally; therefore, M-mode can be erroneous and 2D planimetry is recommended as a preferable method. Left atrial volume measurement by 3D echocardiography has been recently introduced as a natural extension of this trend. We found a better correlation between

LA volume measured by 3D echocardiography and 2D planimetry than that between 3D volume and M-mode diameter (Figure 5.9). As a marker of cardiovascular events, left atrial volume is superior to LA area or diameter, particularly in subjects with sinus rhythm.[10] From LA volume, atrial pump function is also calculated. The LA pump function was reduced when LA was overstretched in our clinical study on hypertrophic cardiomyopathy.

How to image the left atrium for volume measurement

Acquisition
The patient is placed in a left decubital supine position. Left atrial volume acquisition can be made

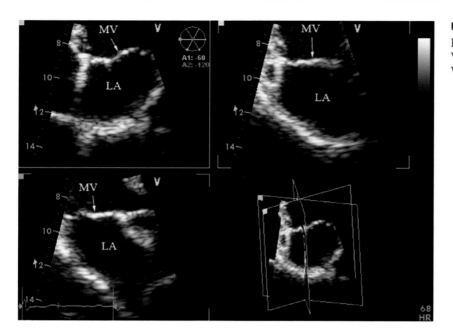

Figure 5.4 Apical view acquired in a patient from three apically rotated views. LA, left atrium; MV, mitral valve.

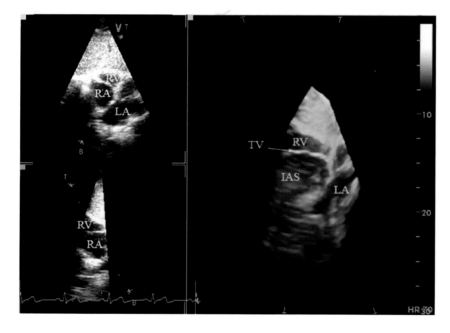

Figure 5.5 Subcostal view and reconstruction of the interatrial septum. LA, left atrium; RA, right atrium, RV, right ventricle; TV, tricuspid valve; IAS, interatrial septum.

from two positions. The first position is from the parasternal view. With this window, the majority of the left atrium is in the ultrasound sector. In our experience of enlarged left atrium, echo dropout may occur in the area of LA roof, even with optimal gain settings.[11] This window is not always appropriate for LA volume measurement, which may explain a weak correlation between MRI and 3D echocardiography.[11] The second position is from the apex, giving a long-axis view of the left atrium. However, even if this scanning position is ideal, the far field limits the spatial resolution and care must be taken when delineating the endocardium for volume measurement. At the present time, there are two ways to determine LA volumes from a 3D volume image,

one with the rotation of apical images (60° apart, as seen in Figure 5.4) and the other with equidistant horizontal slices (9 slices, as seen in Figure 5.10).

Image analysis and structure delineation

The images can be reviewed on-line and off-line. Those corresponding to the largest, the smallest, and before atrial contraction (P wave on the ECG) are manually selected. The endocardial borders of the left atrium are then manually traced on all images for each frame, and integrated by customized software to obtain the real volume from the Simpson's rule. The LAA and the pulmonary veins are excluded from tracing. Atrial stroke volume is given by

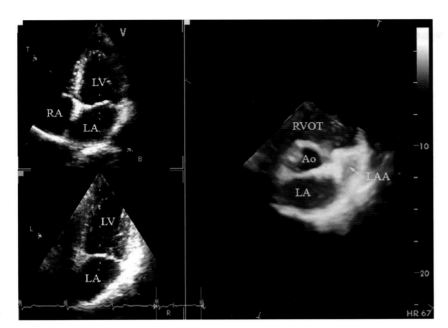

Figure 5.6 Apical view and reconstruction of the left atrial appendage. LA, left atrium; RA, right atrium; LV, left ventricle; Ao, aorta; RVOT, right ventricular outflow tract; LAA, left atrial appendage.

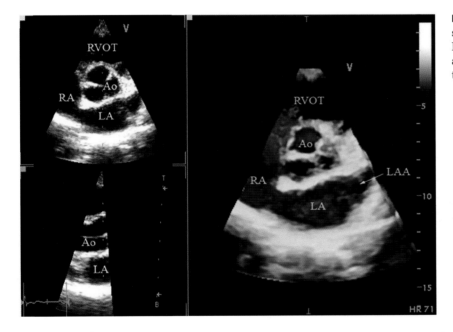

Figure 5.7 Parasternal view and reconstruction of the left atrial appendage. LA, left atrium; RA, right atrium; Ao, aorta; RVOT, right ventricular outflow tract; LAA, left atrial appendage.

(LA volume before atrial contraction – smallest LA volume). Left atrial pump function, expressed in %, is LA stroke volume/LA volume atrial contraction. Conduit and reservoir function are also calculated by these values with the relevant mathematic equations. For a better understanding of LA pathophysiology, the time-varying LA volume curve can be built and analyzed under variable conditions.[11,12] Figure 5.11 shows change in LA volume as a function of time. Table 5.1 gives LA volume and function measured by 3D echocardiography in comparison with variable methods. (Semi-)automatic generation of the LA volume–time curve once the initial manual inputs are done is on the horizon now that the automatic LV volume–time curve is available (Figure 2.13, in Chapter 2).

Normal value and body surface adjustment

Left atrial volume normally increases with age as a consequence of growth and diastolic dysfunction. Table 5.2 gives normal values of LA volume, adjusted to body-surface area.[11,13,14]

Left atrial volume by 3D echocardiography in various diseases

Left atrial enlargement is known to result from pressure overload (mitral stenosis or diastolic dysfunction), volume overload (mitral regurgitation), or intrinsic remodeling/deterioration (atrial fibrillation or myocardial infarction related to left circumflex occlusion). The degree of left atrial enlargement is associated with an adverse prognosis in different

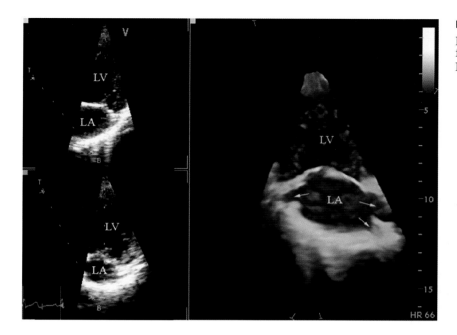

Figure 5.8 Reconstruction of three pulmonary vein inlets (yellow arrows) from an apical imaging. LA, left atrium; LV, left ventricle.

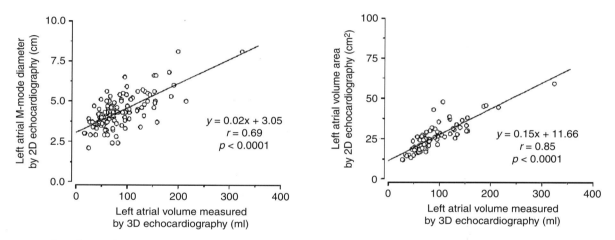

Figure 5.9   Correlation between M-mode LA diameter, 2D LA planimetry, and real-time 3D LA volume.

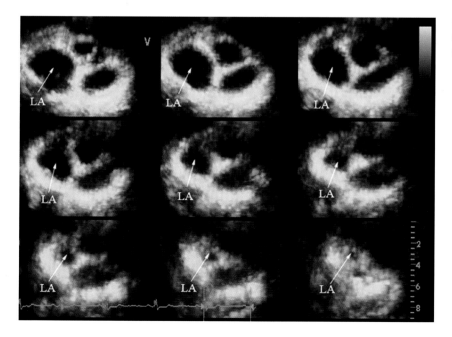

Figure 5.10 In the same beat, the left atrium (LA) is sliced in 9 equidistant cutting planes from the apical view.

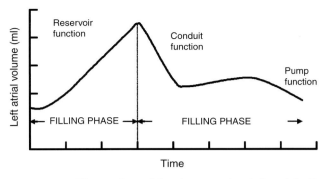

Figure 5.11 Illustration of the time-varying left atrial 3D volume.

clinical settings such as atrial fibrillation, heart failure, stroke, and death. In prediction of cardiovascular events, LA volume is reportedly superior to LA area and diameter.[10] Therefore, LA volume should not be completely ignored in clinical practice any more.

In ischemic disease

In a sheep model of acute ischemia, we experimentally reported that LA volume and function contribution to LV function calculated by 3D echocardiography was better during left anterior descending coronary occlusion than during left

Table 5.1   Left atrial volume measurement by 2D and 3D echocardiography

Reference	Acquisition	Volume derived from	Validation	Main results
Schabelman et al 1981[34]	Parasternal M-mode LA diameter	Cubed method	Angiography	$r = 0.69$
Schabelman et al 1981[34]	Apical 4- and 2-chamber	Biplane area–length	Angiography	$r = 0.86$
Keller et al 2000[35]	Apical 4- and 2-chamber (free-hand)	Disk summation	MRI	$r = 0.90$
Poutanen et al 2000[11]	Parasternal rotation at 18° rotation	Disk summation	MRI	r varying between 0.48 and 0.72
Khankirawatana et al 2002[36]	Apical rotational sweep	Disk summation	No validation	
Bauer et al 2004[17]	Apical	Disk summation	MRI	$r = 0.91$
Jenkins et al 2005[4]	Apical	12 apical rotations with multiplanar Simpson's rule	No validation	No correlation

Table 5.2   Body surface area corrected LA volume

	Body surface area				
	0.5–0.75 m²	0.75–1.0 m²	1.0–1.25 m²	1.25–1.5 m²	>1.5 m²
LA maximum volume (ml)	12.8 ± 2.8	19.1 ± 3.4	25.0 ± 5.8	33.6 ± 6.8	47.8 ± 13.5
LA mid-diastolic volume (ml)	6.2 ± 1.6	9.8 ± 2.0	13.2 ± 3.3	18.6 ± 4.3	27.4 ± 9.0
LA minimum volume (ml)	4.4 ± 1.1	6.7 ± 1.4	8.8 ± 2.4	12.5 ± 3.3	18.2 ± 6.0
LA stroke volume (ml)	1.8 ± 0.8	3.2 ± 1.1	4.3 ± 1.4	6.1 ± 1.7	9.2 ± 4.0

circumflex occlusion.[12] A direct loss of LA contractile units was pathophysiologically implicated in this finding evidenced on the LA pressure–volume relationship (Figure 5.12).

In chronic myocardial infarction, the maximal LA volume has an independent and incremental prognostic value compared with clinical data and conventional measures of LV systolic and diastolic function.[15] LA dilation is the consequence of increased end-diastolic pressure or of direct contractile unit loss as seen in left circumflex occlusion. In ischemic heart disease, therefore, real LA volume measurement by 3D echocardiography may be valuable to evaluate the hemodynamic conditions as well as formulate the prognosis.

In hypertrophic cardiomyopathy

The prevalence of left atrial dilation is variable in patients with hypertrophic cardiomyopathy but is definitely correlated to the severity of the disease.[16] When LA enlargement is present, patients have more frequent cardiovascular events. We found that LA enlargement by 3D echocardiography was related to LV filling pressure, LV outflow tract pressure gradient, and LV wall thickness in patients with hypertrophic cardiomyopathy.[17] We suggested that acting earlier on LA dilation might prevent cardiovascular events in this population.

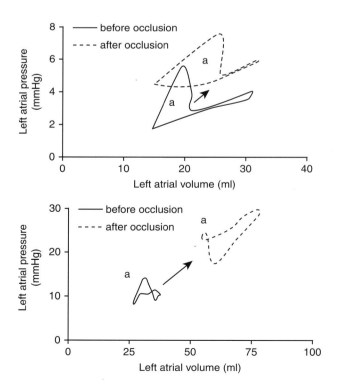

Figure 5.12 Left atrial pressure–volume loops at baseline and during coronary occlusion. Top, during left anterior descending coronary occlusion, atrial function "a" is enhanced. Bottom, during left circumflex coronary occlusion, atrial function "a" is depressed.

THE LEFT ATRIUM IN VARIOUS DISEASES BY 3D ECHOCARDIOGRAPHY

Three-dimensional echocardiography has been used to characterize atrial septal defect and core triatriatum along with left atrial mass and tumor.

Cor triatriatum

Cor triatriatum is a congenital heart disease in which the left atrium is divided into two chambers by a perforated membrane. It has been demonstrated that cor triatriatum is commonly misdiagnosed, confounded with mitral stenosis. When a wide-angled full volume 3D image is to be obtained from apical or parasternal views, the left atrium can be sliced from any plane to differentiate mitral stenosis from cor triatriatum.[18] Three-dimensional navigation and volume-rendered reconstruction visualize the inside of the LA chamber and precisely localize the membrane, its attachment, the size of the opening, and relationships to the pulmonary veins. Three-dimensional echocardiography makes it easy to use Loeffler's classification, relying on the number and size of the openings in the membrane, as well as Marin–Garcia's classification based on the anatomic shape of the accessory LA chamber (diaphragmatic, hour-glass configuration, and tubular).

Atrial septal defect

Nanda et al first imaged interatrial abnormality using 3D TEE.[19] A few years later, Acar et al demonstrated that transthoracic echocardiography was as accurate as transesophageal 3D echocardiography for imaging and sizing atrial septal defects in children.[20] Along with diameter, many different anatomic shapes were described: round, ovoid,

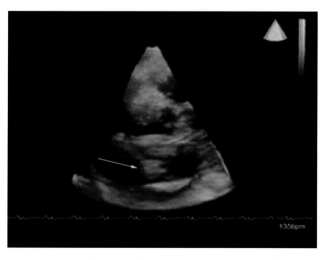

Figure 5.13 Left atrial thrombus (arrow) imaged from a parasternal window.

racket configuration, and multiperforated atrial septal defects. Three-dimensional echocardiography was judged useful to detail the relationship between atrial septal defects and environmental structures such as the aortic root and the tricuspid valve. When the rims surrounding the defect were too small, the transcatheter atrial septal approach was inappropriate for closure. More recently, atrial septal defects have been demonstrated to undergo dynamic changes through the cardiac cycle.[21,22] From those 3D studies, it appeared that a single atrial septal defect, round with good rims and less contractile, was the most appropriate configuration for percutaneous closure.

Tumors and thrombus

Only a few cases of left atrial tumors have been reported in the literature.[23–26] Three-dimensional echocardiography addresses connections and anatomic relations between structures, facilitates volume measurement, and is adapted to follow-up in case of specific therapeutics. In the literature, left atrial tumors were scanned both from the transoesophageal and transthoracic approach.[24,26] For left atrial myxoma, 3D echocardiography navigation easily locates the point of insertion and displays adhesion to multiple regions, whereas 3D reconstruction clarifies whether the tumor adheres to the mitral valve or the left atrium and hems in the left ventricle.[27] Recently, real-time transthoracic 3D echocardiography has been shown to provide a definite diagnosis of myxoma by identifying isolated echolucent areas consistent with hemorrhage/ necrosis by using a section plane of the tumor mass. A patient with a haemangioma showed much more extensive and closely packed echolucencies consistent with a highly vascularized tumor by the live 3D echocardiography.[23]

Generally speaking, real-time transthoracic echocardiography has a poor sensitivity for the detection of left atrial thrombosis until it attains a definite dimension. Again, the TEE approach appears more consistent, but the literature is limited to a few case reports. Rotational 3D echocardiography was employed to evidence large LAA thrombosis, but recently Ieva et al have reported the usefulness of live 3D transthoracic echocardiography in a typical case of large thrombus floating in the left atrium.[7,12,28] We report here an example of LA thrombus after the resection of LA posterior wall (Figure 5.12). The thrombus could be easily viewed from the sides along with its morphology and the site of attachment. In this case, by cropping the 3D images sequentially, the degree and extent of lysis within the thrombus, which may have potential therapeutic and prognostic implications, could be comprehensively assessed after the anticoagulation was started. Finally, real-time 3D echocardiography provided information of thrombus mobility, which has also prognostic implications.

THREE-DIMENSIONAL ECHOCARDIOGRAPHY-GUIDED THERAPY IN THE LEFT ATRIUM ENVIRONMENT

Live 3D echocardiography provides in a few seconds a reliable reconstruction of variable LA surgical views using transthoracic or epicardial echocardiography. Prior to operation, surgeons may have relevant information to design and to limit the exploratory phase of the procedure. During the procedure, 3D echocardiography may be essential in monitoring valve and congenital heart disease repairs and, if necessary, in assessing hemodynamic failure. Only a few centers make use of 3D echocardiography to monitor patients and procedures.

One of the strongest indications for intraoperative 3D echocardiography is 'line' atrial septal defect closure monitored by epicardial real-time 3D echocardiography without cardiopulmonary bypass.[29] In an animal experiment, Suematsu et al found a good agreement between atrial septal defect planimetry by 3D and true anatomic area.[29] Furthermore, they found 3D echocardiography to be quite useful to assess the spatial relationship between the atrial septal defect and peripheral structures such as the tricuspid valve and the coronary sinus. Three-dimensional echocardiography properly monitored atrial septal defect closure and assisted in positioning of intravascular devices. For multiple atrial septal defects, 3D TEE provided in one single view the size, configuration, and the relationship of the defects to adjacent structures.[30] This 3D visualization of multiple atrial septal defects was particularly useful to select the appropriate occluder and to ascertain complete closure.

A fascinating application of 3D echocardiography in combination with image fusion techniques is pulmonary vein ablation in the setting of atrial fibrillation (AF). To date, several techniques are used for AF ablation, but no general consensus exists as to which technique is the most effective between 3D intracardiac echocardiography, computed tomography, and MRI. However, 3D echocardiography has many advantages over the other techniques. First, the transseptal puncture can be easily guided by intracardiac echocardiography. Second, 3D echocardiography provides a unique dynamic view of the pulmonary veins from real-time transesophageal echocardiography or phased-array transducer (ACU-NAV, Siemens) positioned in the right atrium.[31] More recently, a 9-French prototype catheter with incorporated intracardiac 3D echocardiography has been tested to image the ablation.[32] Three-dimensional reconstruction is less studied except one publication that correlated outcome of flutter ablation and isthmus anatomical variants particularly due to Eustachian ridge peculiarities.[33] Advantages of 3D echocardiography are 4-fold:

(1) It precisely identifies the true border of the pulmonary vein antrum.
(2) All the pulmonary veins are electrically isolated at the level of the antrum.
(3) It avoids the risk of PV stenosis by ablating outside the antrum.
(4) It minimizes the risk of other complications, such as perforation and stroke, by direct visualization during transseptal access and radiofrequency ablation.

Overall, exceedingly long fluoroscopy times for ablation procedures may be overcome in the near future by 3D echocardiography i.e. methods, especially by the recently introduced real-time TEE 3D echocardiography.

For percutaneous LAA occlusion, 3D echocardiography is not yet used. Left atrial thrombus is a contraindication to percutaneous mitral valve procedures (commissurotomy of mitral stenosis or edge to edge repair of mitral regurgitation). Preprocedural use of 3D echocardiography to exclude this finding might be credited with a reduction in the occurrence of complications.

CONCLUSION

Three-dimensional echocardiography has the ability to assess left atrial volume and function more accurately than 2D imaging. By freely navigating in a volume dataset and giving an *en face* view of any volume-rendered reconstruction, 3D echocardiography offers the true inside and outside vision of the LA. Recently developed on-line LA reconstruction is one of the most fascinating techniques helping surgeons and interventional cardiologists to deliver the best understanding and management therapy for cardiac patients with LA abnormalities.

REFERENCES

1. Rossi A, Zardini P, Marino P. Modulation of left atrial function by ventricular filling impairment. Heart Fail Rev 2000; 5: 325–31.

2. Tabata T, Oki T, Yamada H et al. Role of left atrial appendage in left atrial reservoir function as evaluated by left atrial appendage clamping during cardiac surgery. Am J Cardiol 1998; 81: 327–32.

3. Bauer F, Verdonck A, Schuster I et al. Left atrial appendage function analyzed by tissue Doppler imaging in mitral stenosis: effect of afterload reduction after mitral valve commissurotomy. J Am Soc Echocardiogr 2005; 18: 934–9.

4. Jenkins C, Bricknell K, Marwick TH. Use of real-time three-dimensional echocardiography to measure left atrial volume: comparison with other echocardiographic techniques. J Am Soc Echocardiogr 2005; 18: 991–7.

5. Valocik G, Kamp O, Mihciokur M et al. Assessment of the left atrial appendage mechanical function by three-dimensional echocardiography. Eur J Echocardiogr 2002; 3: 207–13.

6. Agoston I, Xie T, Tiller FL, Rahman AM, Ahmad M. Assessment of left atrial appendage by live three-dimensional echocardiography: early experience and comparison with transesophageal echocardiography. Echocardiography 2006; 23: 127–32.

7. Khan GN, Dairywala IT, Liu Z et al. Three-dimensional echocardiography of left atrial appendage thrombus. Echocardiography 2001; 18: 163–6.

8. Tsang TS, Barnes ME, Bailey KR et al. Left atrial volume: important risk marker of incident atrial fibrillation in 1655 older men and women. Mayo Clin Proc 2001; 76: 467–75.

9. Khankirawatana B, Khankirawatana S, Porter T. How should left atrial size be reported? Comparative assessment with use of multiple echocardiographic methods. Am Heart J 2004; 147: 369–74.

10. Tsang TS, Abhayaratna WP, Barnes ME et al. Prediction of cardiovascular outcomes with left atrial size: is volume superior to area or diameter? J Am Coll Cardiol 2006; 47: 1018–23.

11. Poutanen T, Ikonen A, Vainio P, Jokinen E, Tikanoja T. Left atrial volume assessed by transthoracic three dimensional echocardiography and magnetic resonance imaging: dynamic changes during the heart cycle in children. Heart 2000; 83: 537–42.

12. Bauer F, Jones M, Qin JX et al. Quantitative analysis of left atrial function during left ventricular ischemia with and without left atrial ischemia: a real-time 3-dimensional echocardiographic study. J Am Soc Echocardiogr 2005; 18: 795–801.

13. Kawai J, Tanabe K, Wang CL et al. Comparison of left atrial size by freehand scanning three-dimensional echocardiography and two-dimensional echocardiography. Eur J Echocardiogr 2004; 5: 18–24.

14. Poutanen T, Jokinen E, Sairanen H, Tikanoja T. Left atrial and left ventricular function in healthy children and young adults assessed by three dimensional echocardiography. Heart 2003; 89: 544–9.

15. Moller JE, Hillis GS, Oh JK et al. Left atrial volume: a powerful predictor of survival after acute myocardial infarction. Circulation 2003; 107: 2207–12.

16. Yang H, Woo A, Monakier D et al. Enlarged left atrial volume in hypertrophic cardiomyopathy: a marker for disease severity. J Am Soc Echocardiogr 2005; 18: 1074–82.

17. Bauer F, Shiota T, White RD et al. Determinant of left atrial dilation in patients with hypertrophic cardiomyopathy: a

real-time 3-dimensional echocardiographic study. J Am Soc Echocardiogr 2004; 17: 968–75.

18. Jacobs A, Weinert LC, Goonewardena S, Gomberg-Maitland M, Lang RM. Three-dimensional transthoracic echocardiography to evaluate cor triatriatum in the adult. J Am Soc Echocardiogr 2006; 19: 468 e1–4.

19. Nanda NC, Ansingkar K, Espinal M et al. Transesophageal three-dimensional echo assessment of sinus venosus atrial septal defect. Echocardiography 1999; 16: 835–7.

20. Acar P, Dulac Y, Roux D et al. Comparison of transthoracic and transesophageal three-dimensional echocardiography for assessment of atrial septal defect diameter in children. Am J Cardiol 2003; 91: 500–2.

21. Xie MX, Fang LY, Wang XF et al. Assessment of atrial septal defect area changes during cardiac cycle by live three-dimensional echocardiography. J Cardiol 2006; 47: 181–7.

22. Handke M, Schafer DM, Muller G et al. Dynamic changes of atrial septal defect area: new insights by three-dimensional volume-rendered echocardiography with high temporal resolution. Eur J Echocardiogr 2001; 2: 46–51.

23. Borges AC, Witt C, Bartel T et al. Preoperative two- and three-dimensional transesophageal echocardiographic assessment of heart tumors. Ann Thorac Surg 1996; 61: 1163–7.

24. Salustri A, Roelandt J. Images in cardiovascular medicine. Left atrial myxoma visualized by transesophageal rotoplane echocardiographic computed tomography. Circulation 1995; 91: 2290.

25. Greco C, Romano P, Di Segni M, Prati PL. Three-dimensional transesophageal echocardiographic evaluation of a left atrial myxoma. G Ital Cardiol 1998; 28: 193.

26. Mehmood F, Nanda NC, Vengala S et al. Live three-dimensional transthoracic echocardiographic assessment of left atrial tumors. Echocardiography 2005; 22: 137–43.

27. Harada T, Ohtaki E, Sumiyoshi T, Hosoda S. Successful three-dimensional reconstruction using transesophageal echocardiography in a patient with a left atrial myxoma. Jpn Heart J 2001; 42: 789–92.

28. Ieva R, Correale M, Pellegrino PL, Di Biase M. Three-dimensional transthoracic echocardiographic visualization of a voluminous left atrial thrombus. Echocardiography 2006; 23: 81–2.

29. Suematsu Y, Martinez JF, Wolf BK et al. Three-dimensional echo-guided beating heart surgery without cardiopulmonary bypass: atrial septal defect closure in a swine model. J Thorac Cardiovasc Surg 2005; 130: 1348–57.

30. Cao Q, Radtke W, Berger F, Zhu W, Hijazi ZM. Transcatheter closure of multiple atrial septal defects. Initial results and value of two- and three-dimensional transoesophageal echocardiography. Eur Heart J 2000; 21: 941–7.

31. Pua EC, Idriss SF, Wolf PD, Smith SW. Real-time 3D transesophageal echocardiography. Ultrason Imaging 2004; 26: 217–32.

32. Gentry KL, Smith SW. Integrated catheter for 3-D intracardiac echocardiography and ultrasound ablation. IEEE Trans Ultrason Ferroelectr Freq Control 2004; 51: 800–8.

33. Scaglione M, Caponi D, Di Donna P et al. Typical atrial flutter ablation outcome: correlation with isthmus anatomy using intracardiac echo 3D reconstruction. Europace 2004; 6: 407–17.

34. Schabelman S, Schiller NB, Silverman NH, Povt TA. Left atrial volume estimation by two-dimensional echocardiography. Cathet Cardiovasc Diagn 1981; 7: 165–78.

35. Keller AM, Gopal AS, King DL. Left and right atrial volume by freehand three-dimensional echocardiography: in vivo validation using magnetic resonance imaging. Eur J Echocardiogr 2000; 1: 55–65.

36. Khankirawatana B, Khankirawatana S, Lof J, Porter TR. Left atrial volume determination by three-dimensional echocardiography reconstruction: validation and application of a simplified technique. J Am Soc Echocardiogr 2002; 15: 1051–6.

6 Valvular Heart Disease: Mitral Valve; Mitral Regurgitation

Takahiro Shiota

The etiology of mitral regurgitation (MR) consists of degenerative changes (mitral valve prolapse), flail (Figure 6.1), rheumatic valve disease, infective endocarditis, dilated mitral annulus, and restrictive motion due to papillary muscle dysfunction with left ventricular (LV) wall motion abnormality, so-called functional MR (Figure 6.2), congenital cleft of the anterior leaflet (Figure 6.3), and radiation.

Conventional two-dimensional (2D) echocardiographic methods, including transesophageal echocardiography (TEE), can demonstrate such anatomic abnormalities, causing MR in most patients. Severity of MR can be also determined by 2D echocardiography. There are quite a few 2D echocardiographic methods for determining the severity of MR, including the color Doppler jet area, proximal isovelocity surface area (PISA) or flow convergence (FC) method, vena contracta (proximal jet width) method and the pulmonary venous flow pattern method.[1–9]

METHODS TO DETERMINE MR SEVERITY

Color jet area method

Many 2D echocardiographic methods for assessing the severity of MR have been proposed and published in a variety of cardiology and ultrasound journals. Among them, the color Doppler regurgitant jet area method is most widely used for judging the severity of MR.[1,2] This visual method is historically the first one and, most importantly, is very simple (Figure 6.4).

In a previous study,[2] the best correlation with angiography was obtained when the maximal MR jet area (MJA) was expressed as a percentage of the left atrial area (LAA) obtained in the same plane. The maximum MJA/LAA was under 20% in 34 of 36 patients with angiographic grade I MR, between 20% and 40% in 17 of 18 patients with grade II MR, and over 40% in 26 of 28 patients with severe MR. Another study,[1] which also used angiography

as a gold standard, demonstrated that an MJA greater than 8 cm^2 predicted severe MR with a sensitivity of 82% and specificity of 94%, whereas an MJA less than 4 cm^2 predicted mild MR with a sensitivity and specificity of 85% and 75%, respectively. All patients with an average jet area greater than 8 cm^2 manifested severe MR. In this study, the authors also reported that the ratio of MJA/LAA provided similar sensitivity or specificity: MJA/LAA > 40% predicts severe MR with a sensitivity of 73% and specificity of 92%; MJA/LAA < 20% predicts mild MR with a sensitivity of 65% and specificity of 93%. When the enlarged LA area is 32 cm^2 in MR patients, 8 cm^2 is calculated as 40% of LAA. Thus, the absolute color jet area or the ratio of MR jet area to LA area can be used to grade the severity of MR.

The aliasing velocity (Nyquest limit) is one of the most important factors when applying this popular method, and should be used at 50–60 cm/s.[10] Multiplane 2D views, including parasternal long/short-axis and apical views, should be used to image MR jets. However, this color Doppler method cannot be properly used in certain patients, including those with artificial valves because of significant sound attenuation. Thus, in such patients, TEE has to be employed to evaluate the severity of MR. However, this jet area depends on many mechanical factors such as pulse repetition frequency, aliasing velocity, imaging field, color gain, priority of tissue and color imaging. Because of these factors, especially closeness of the imaging and less attenuation of the ultrasound, TEE may overestimate the jet area as compared to TTE imaging of MR color jet.[11] As a matter of fact, in a previous study comparing valvular regurgitant severity by TTE and TEE, 6 patients of 13 with moderate regurgitation judged by TTE were graded as severe by TEE. Even mild or none by TTE were graded as severe by TEE in this study.[11]

Therefore, one cannot apply the criteria for TTE when TEE is used for imaging. Also, an eccentric jet or wall impinging jet appears to be smaller than a

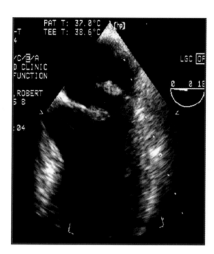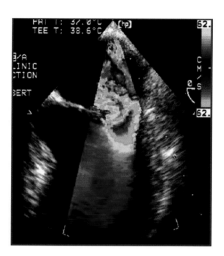

Figure 6.1   An example of transesophageal echocardiography from a patient with severe MR due to the flail of the posterior leaflet.

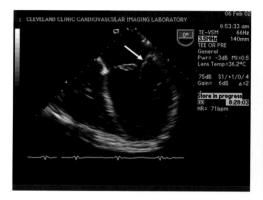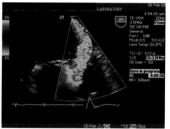

Figure 6.2   An example of transesophageal echocardiography from a patient with severe MR due to the restrictive motion of the posterior leaflet (arrow). The regurgitant jet is eccentric and directed posteriorly. Note a large flow convergence towards the regurgitant orifice.

central jet area even when the regurgitant volume is the same as that of a central jet. In addition, there was only weak correlation between the jet area and the regurgitant volumes in previous 2D echocardiographic studies.[3] Thus, an eccentric, wall-impinging jet swirling in the LA is considered to be severe irrespective of the jet area according to the recommendations from the American Society of Echocardiography.[10] 3D echocardiography may provide more insight in this field because it will demonstrate the entire jet extension without requiring multiple planes or mental reconstruction. It can also determine the absolute regurgitant volume of the complex jet, as will be discussed later.

PISA or flow convergence method (Figure 6.5)

Major advantages of a newer color Doppler echo method, the so-called PISA or FC method, over the color jet area method are as follows. First, this new method is not influenced by color gain. Thus, the operator can increase color gain as much as required

to see the FC surface. Second, this method is not affected by the eccentricity of the MR jet. Once the PISA or FC is optimized, the severity of MR can be judged irrespective of pattern or size of jet extension. More importantly, this new method can provide a quantitative assessment of regurgitant volume and regurgitant orifice area, while the color jet area method cannot. Even when we do not apply a quantitative assessment of valvular regurgitation, the maximal size of FC aliasing distance may be sufficient to judge MR severity. When one does not see FC larger than 4 mm at 40 cm/s, the regurgitation would be trivial or at most mild (or calculated regurgitant orifice area, ROA < 0.2 cm^2). When we see FC larger than 8 mm at the aliasing velocity > 50 cm/s (or ROA > 0.4 cm^2), the regurgitation is severe. All regurgitations in between are deemed moderate.

This 2D FC method is easy to apply and thus is recommended when one only needs to judge the severity of valvular regurgitation semiquantitatively. However these 2D FC methods assume a hemispheric shape of FC to assess MR severity, and thus have limitations when the FC shape is not hemispheric.

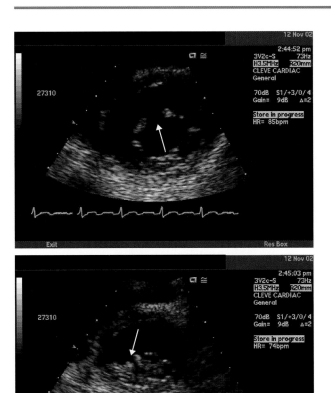

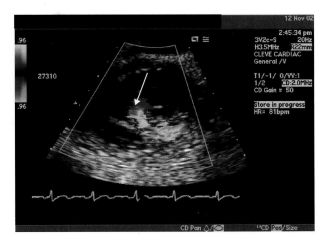

Figure 6.3 An example of a transthoracic echocardiogram from a patient with moderately severe MR due to a cleft of the anterior leaflet. The upper left panel shows a diastolic phase and the bottom a systolic one. Arrows show the cleft.

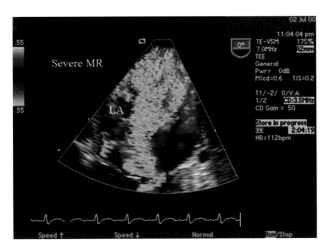

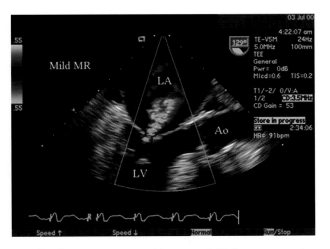

Figure 6.4 Pre (left panel) and post (right panel) repairs of the mitral valve in a patient with severe MR due to a restrictive motion of the mitral valve leaflets and dilated annulus. Note the remarkable reduction of the color jet area of the regurgitation after the repair.

3D color Doppler echocardiography, which is now available, can overcome this limitation, leading to more accurate assessment of MR severity. This new method may change the concept of the FC grading system, as will be discussed later.

Vena contracta (proximal jet width) method (Figure 6.6)

This method is another echo/Doppler technique for grading and quantifying the severity of MR. The color

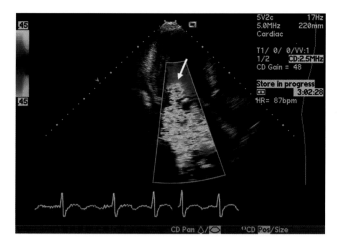

Figure 6.5 An example of the flow convergence (arrow) towards the mitral regurgitant orifice or proximal isovelocity surface area from a patient with severe MR due to mitral valve prolapse.

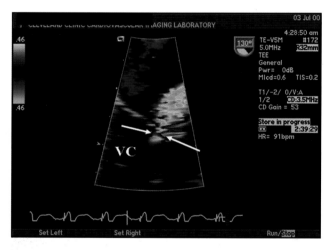

Figure 6.6 An example of vena contracta imaging (VC, arrows) from a patient with mild MR by TEE.

Doppler imaged vena contracta (VC) is defined as the connection of the regurgitant jet and the flow acceleration, as seen in Figure 6.6. In order to find VC, one may start to see FC and look for a regurgitant jet while still keeping the FC image on the monitor. In this manner, one can find the connection between the FC and regurgitant jet, which is a color-imaged VC. A width of the vena contracta less than 0.3 cm is considered to be mild MR, and equal to or greater than 0.7 cm severe. It is still not quite as easy as the jet area or FC method in day to day practice, probably because of the technical difficulty in demonstrating a clear VC. However, when a high-resolution image of VC is available, especially in TEE as seen in Figure 6.6, this may be quite a useful alternative to the FC and color jet area method.

In a clinical TEE study, a diameter > 0.55 cm was suggestive of severe MR, although the authors did not express their 'regurgitant jet width at its

origin' as VC. 3D echocardiography can potentially provide a more precise location, shape, and size of VC when real-time TEE 3D echocardiography becomes available.

Pulmonary venous flow (Figure 6.7)

Pulmonary venous flow patterns recorded by the pulsed Doppler method are another aid for grading the severity of MR. In one of the earliest clinical studies, 26 (93%) of 28 patients with severe regurgitation by transesophageal color flow mapping had reversed systolic flow. The sensitivity of reversed systolic flow in detecting severe 4+ mitral regurgitation by transesophageal color flow mapping was 93% and the specificity was 100%. However, this flow pattern may be influenced by the location of the sampling site, or selection of the four pulmonary veins interrogated, and left ventricular performance.

Other echo indices for judging the severity of MR

As a result of volume overloading, in patients with severe MR, LV and LA size are increased and early diastolic transmitral flow (E wave) velocity is also increased. Dense CW Doppler signal of MR is also expected in severe MR. Such echo indices should be sought and systematically assessed in the final judgment of the severity of MR.

APPLICATION OF 3D ECHOCARDIOGRAPHY

Then what would be the clinical value of 3D echocardiography in patients with MR? First of all, one can see the mitral valve in a way most natural to the human senses, the so-called *en face* or surgical view (Figures 6.8–6.12). No 2D echocardiography can show these images. For example, see Figure 6.8: the location and extension/volume of the posterior leaflet prolapse are easily fathomed by this *en face* view.

Medical students and patients along with cardiac surgeons can appreciate this presentation and anatomic abnormality of the mitral valve much better than those made by 2D echocardiography, which requires multiple views, mental reconstruction, and many years of experience. Even the best echocardiologist with state of the art 2D equipment is not able to discern the exact anatomy of the mitral valve as well as this 3D figure demonstrates.

TRANSESOPHAGEAL 3D RECONSTRUCTION

The advantage of having a view of the entire valve with the use of TEE with 3D reconstruction has been

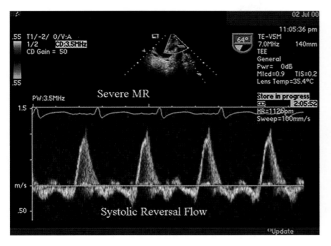

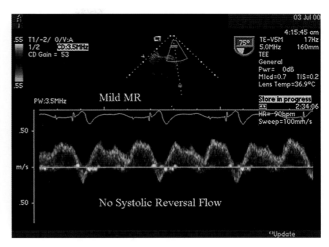

Figure 6.7 Comparison of pulmonary venous flow pattern between pre (left panel) and post (right panel) repairs of the mitral valve in a patient with severe MR. Note the remarkable change of the pattern (see text) after the repair. From the same patient as Figure 6.4.

repeatedly reported.[12–16] In a previous study, TEE with 3D reconstruction was used in 91 patients with severe MR due to mitral valve prolapse, and the location and extent of the prolapse by echo were compared to the surgical status. The volume of the prolapsing leaflet was calculated and compared to the volume of resected tissue whenever a repair was attempted. There was an excellent correlation between the echocardiographic localization of the prolapse and surgical inspection, and between the volume of prolapsing and surgically resected tissue ($r = 0.94$, $p < 0.0001$). The authors concluded that the 3D reconstruction echo method allowed a precise localization and an accurate quantification of the prolapsing portion of the leaflets. Reconstruction TEE 3D echocardiography, therefore, can provide refinements in the surgical planning of mitral valve repair and in the selection of candidates for this intervention.

Regrettably, this valuable method is not widely used yet. This can be explained, in my opinion, by its technical difficulties, including suboptimal gating, synchronization due to the motion of patients and the TEE probe during sequential 2D imaging, and also by cumbersome reconstruction techniques. A few cardiologists (even among echo specialists) can actually obtain satisfactory *en face* mitral valve images like Figure 6.8. As far as I know, few cardiac centers would be able to implement this valuable 3D method in clinical practice despite its potential value. The recently reported new real-time 3D TEE is our hope to overcome such limitations.[17,18] Once such methods are introduced in the operating and cardiac catheterization rooms, dramatic changes may take place in the monitoring of surgical and percutaneous procedures.

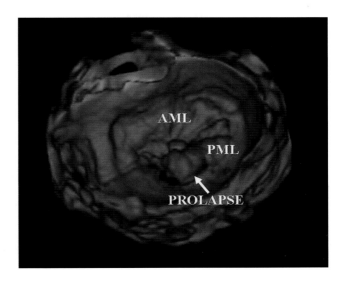

Figure 6.8 A surgical view of a mitral valve proplapse (middle scallop) AML: anterior mitral leaflet, PML: posterior mitral leaflet.

TRANSTHORACIC REAL-TIME 3D ECHOCARDIOGRAPHY

As for transthoracic real-time 3D echocardiography, higher-resolution methods are now available from multiple vendors. This newer type transthoracic real-time 3D echocardiography currently requires ECG gating for obtaining the entire mitral valve from the apex. Nonetheless, it is still much easier to apply and more consistent and reliable than any previous 3D echocardiographic method. For example, Figures 6.9 and 6.10 were obtained as part of a clinical examination in our echo laboratory. It took our sonographer an additional 5 minutes

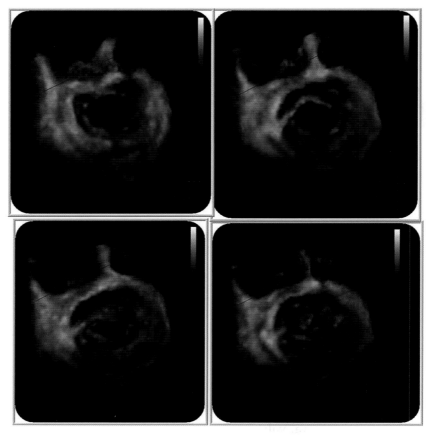

Figure 6.9 Temporal changes in 3D *en face* view of the mitral valve. Note the cleft of the anterior leaflet (right lower panel).

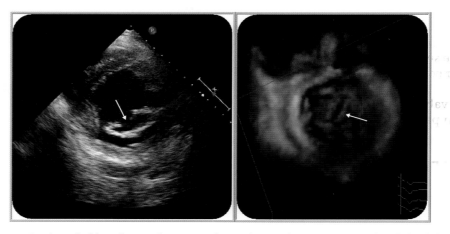

Figure 6.10 2D short-axis view (left) and transthoracic echocardiography 3D images of a cleft of the anterior leaflet. Note the striking difference in the presentation of the cleft.

approximately for acquiring 3D imaging and another 5 minutes for me to evaluate it. When I started the study of 3D echocardiography about a decade ago, I had to wait until the following morning to obtain just one 3D reconstruction image. The result was almost always unsatisfactory, making me constantly disappointed. I was convinced at that time that 3D echocardiography must become easy, handy, and user-friendly.

Finally, the eagerly anticipated, new real-time transthoracic 3D echo is here. Figure 6.9 demonstrates time sequential changes in *en face* views of a mitral valve from our routine 3D studies. When one compares the 3D *en face* view with a corresponding 2D short-axis view side by side (Figure 6.10), the difference is striking. While 2D echo can show a part of the cleft of the anterior leaflet in this patient, the 3D *en face* view can demonstrate the *entire*

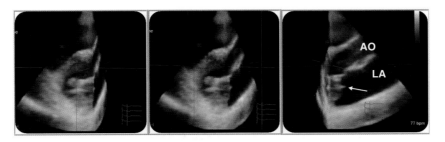

Figure 6.11   Rotated 3D views of a flail of the posterior leaflet. The exact location of the flail is detected (arrow).

cleft, which runs obliquely from the tip of the anterior leaflet towards the aorta-mitral continuation (Figure 6.10). In our laboratory, the mitral valve is almost always successfully visualized in everyday clinical practice because of its handiness and user-friendly software.

In another patient with flail and severe prolapse of the posterior leaflet, one can see the exact location of the flail of the posterior leaflet (slightly lateral side of the mid-posterior scallop) by rotating the 3D views, as seen in Figure 6.11. Confidence about the exact location of the flail in this patient increased when 3D echo was analyzed after routine 2D echo examination. Our surgeon confirmed this 3D finding when he repaired this mitral valve flail and prolapse.

This confirmation of the location of the 2D plane by 3D echo is analogous to the use of 2D echo for locating the M-mode curser line. In the olden days, we often felt very assured when the placement of the M-mode curser line was confirmed by viewing the corresponding 2D imaging. It is no wonder that the superiority of real-time 3D echocardiography over conventional 2D echo methods was reported multiple times[19,20] in analyzing the anatomy of the mitral valve and replaced artificial valve (Figure 6.12) in patients with MR.

COLOR DOPPLER 3D ECHOCARDIOGRAPHY IN MR

The advent of color Doppler 3D has allowed us to have hitherto unforeseen images of MR jet and flow convergence in patients with MR.

MR jet visualization

For example, in a patient with status/post mitral valve replacement, 2D TEE showed a wall impinging jet as seen in Figure 6.13 (upper panel). The size of the jet was small and thin in all 2D TEE views. However, our TEE 3D reconstruction method disclosed a much larger paravalvular MR jet, as seen in Figure 6.13 (lower panels). The MR jet was adhering to the wall very strongly, and stretched

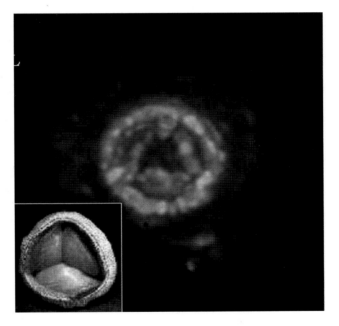

Figure 6.12   Carpentier–Edward tissue valve (actual picture in the lower left) and 3D image. 2D echocardiography cannot demonstrate all three leaflets in a view.

towards the LA curved wall. It was impossible to demonstrate the entire jet by conventional 2D TEE. This is why a wall-impinging eccentric jet should be considered to be severe even when its area is relatively small (remember the 2D criteria of 'severe' by the ASE recommendation).

The 3D *en face* images also demonstrated the exact location of the paravalvular leakage, which was also impossible to fathom by 2D TEE. Or, it may be possible to do guesswork, but not possible to be absolutely certain by any 2D echo method. As seen in this case, color Doppler 3D echocardiography can reveal unique views and the actual volume of the MR jet, which cannot be appreciated by multiple 2D echo views.[21,22] Some enthusiastic investigators even measured the volume of 3D MR jets and reported that it was a better parameter for assessing the severity of MR than the 2D color jet area method.[21,22] However, again, this TEE 3D reconstruction method is still labor intensive and not user-friendly. Thus it is not yet applied widely in clinical practice.

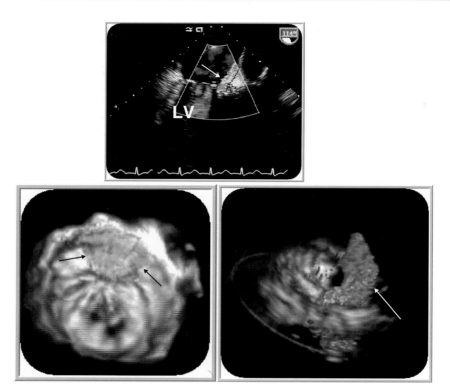

Figure 6.13 A paravalvular MR in a patient with status post mitral valve replacement. Conventional 2D transesophageal echocardiography (TEE) showed a thin, relatively small MR jet (upper panel (white arrow)). In contrast, a wall-adherent curved large MR jet is visualized by the TEE 3D reconstruction method (lower panels (black and white arrows)).

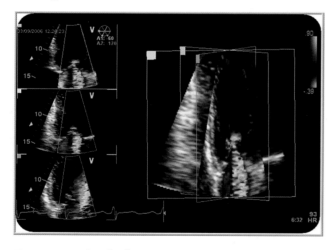

Figure 6.14 A mitral regurgitant MR jet is seen in three different apical plane views taken at the same time.

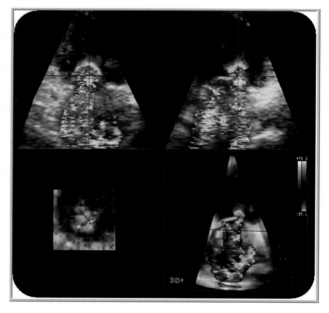

Figure 6.15 Severe functional mitral regurgitation imaged by color Doppler 3D echo. Note that the proximal isovelocity surface area (PISA) shape and size are different among these images. Mitral regurgitation appears to pass through the valve coaptation (lower left panel).

On the other hand, as mentioned above, handy transthoracic real-time 3D echo with color Doppler capability is now available, as seen in Figures 6.14– 6.17. Figure 6.14 demonstrates multiple 2D planes obtained simultaneously in a patient with functional MR. These are not 3D volume data, only multiple 2D plane data. The simultaneous, multiple plane function of 3D echo systems are actually useful, especially when one needs to know the exact location, size, and shape of PISA.

The image quality is the same as that of conventional 2D echocardiography.

When a 3D volume set is acquired, one can have arbitrary desirable 2D planes from the 3D volume, as

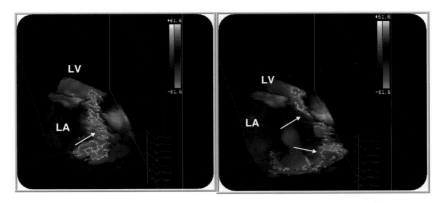

Figure 6.16 MR jet extensions viewed from the left atrium (LA) in two different cardiac phases. Note that the jet extension (arrows) changes during the cardiac cycle. LV; left ventricle.

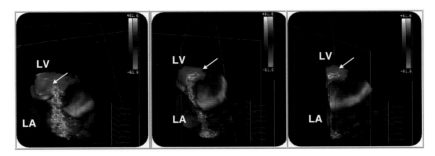

Figure 6.17 Rotated views of a PISA. Note the rounded shape of PISA in the left panel and elongated shape in the right panel. LA; Left atrium, LV; left ventricle.

seen in Figure 6.15. The image quality of Figure 6.15 is not as good as that of Figure 6.14 because Figure 6.15 comes from an entire 3D volume dataset while Figure 6.14 does not. However, any desirable short-axis plane can be obtained, as seen in the left lower panel. Such a short-axis plane is not possible from the apex by the multiple 2D plane method, as in Figure 6.14. This short-axis plane can show both the anterior and posterior leaflet and the MR through these two leaflets. From the 3D volume set, reconstruction of the entire MR jet and PISA is also available, as seen in Figures 6.16 and 6.17. When MR jet extension is complicated, the entire jet cannot be seen in a single 2D view.

Only 3D color Doppler can capture and demonstrate the entire jet to evaluate its direction and volume. When an MR jet is examined carefully, often the direction and extension of the jet are dynamically changing, as seen in Figure 6.16. Again, only color 3D echocardiography can demonstrate such dynamic changes in the MR jet.

PISA visualization and quantification

In Figure 6.17, PISA shape looks like a hemisphere from a vertical or apical view, while in a horizontal (parallel to the mitral annular plane) view, the same PISA looks very elongated. Such recognition

of PISA is not possible by conventional 2D echocardiography. Since the conventional 2D PISA method assumes a hemispheric shape for PISA (like that of Figure 6.17, vertical or apical view), 3D color Doppler is indispensable for assessing PISA and MR severity when PISA shape is not hemispheric (Figure 6.15). As seen, 3D color Doppler methods now can demonstrate the 3D shape of PISA and allow us to correct erroneous calculations of the MR orifice area or regurgitant volume.

QUANTITATIVE 3D ECHOCARDIOGRAPHY IN AN MR PATIENT

Three-dimensional echocardiography with color Doppler capability now allows us to attempt quantitative assessment of MR volumes and absolute LV volume and function in an MR patient.

Direct determination of MR volume

After acquiring 3D PISA images from a patient with MR, one can check the shape of PISA from multiple views. If it is not a hemisphere, one can change it by lowering aliasing velocities.[23,24] When the 3D shape of flow convergence is close enough to a hemisphere, the regurgitant volume can be calculated[24]

A

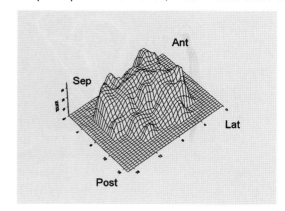

B

Spatial velocity distribution

LVOT: Spatial peak = 40.7 cm/s, mean = 20.5 ± 8.1 cm/s

Figure 6.18 (A) Color 3D presentation of the LVOT velocity profile. (B) Spatial velocity distribution of LVOT flow from the color-coded image in (A). Integration of this velocity information over time will provide LVOT stroke volume without any assumptions of velocity profile.

as $2\pi R^2 \times V \times VTI/Vmax$, where V is the aliasing velocity, in cm/s. Regurgitant orifice area (ROA) is calculated as $2\pi R^2 \times V/Vmax$, where R is maximal aliasing distance from the orifice, in cm, and Vmax is the peak velocity of CW velocity, in cm/s. The duration of the maximal flow rate is calculated as the ratio of velocity time integral to the peak velocity of the regurgitant flow (VTI/Vmax). For example, in a patient with MR when the maximal aliasing distance R = 1.0 cm at the aliasing velocity V = 40 cm/s, and VTI = 100 cm, Vmax = 500 cm/s, ROA is calculated as $2 \times 3.14 \times 1 \times 1 \times 40/500 = 0.5$ cm^2, and regurgitant volume is calculated as $2 \times 3.14 \times 1 \times 1 \times 40 \times 100/500 = 50$ ml.

When the shape of PISA is not a hemisphere, despite the maximal change of the aliasing velocity as in Figure 6.17, more realistic mathematic assumptions such as a curved hemi-ellipsoidal geometry should be applied for determining the PISA area and MR volume. Three-dimensional color Doppler is quite valuable to determine the correctness of using a simple hemispheric PISA method. One can cross-check MR volumes using other 3D echocardiographic method as follows.

Indirect determination of MR volume

MR volumes can be indirectly calculated as the difference between 3D-derived LV end-diastolic volume (EDV), 3D LV end-systolic volume (ESV), and the left ventricular outflow tract (LVOT) stroke volume. As seen in Chapter 2, absolute LV volumes can be determined by real-time transthoracic 3D echocardiography and thus LVEDV − LVESV can be calculated with ease.

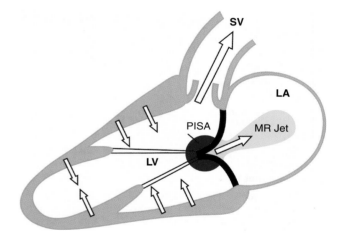

Figure 6.19 Schema of quantitative analysis of MR volume by 3D echocardiography with color Doppler capability. (LV end diastolic volume − LV end systolic volume) by 3D = MR volume by PISA + LVOT Stroke volume (SV). Thus, MR volume = (LV end diastolic volume − LV end systolic volume) − SV (see text in detail).

On the other hand, 3D color Doppler coded velocity information applied on the LVOT (Figures 6.18(A) and (B)) can be integrated over the systolic duration to provide LVOT stroke volume.[25–27] As for this LVOT stroke volume, one can, of course, calculate it using the conventional quantitative Doppler method (3.14 × LVOT diameter × LVOT diameter/4 × VTI of the LVOT velocity). For example, when LVOT diameter = 2.0 cm and VTI of LVOT velocity = 10 cm, then LVOT stroke volume would be $6.28 \times 1 \times 1 \times 10 = 62.8$ ml by this method. However, this 2D conventional pulsed Doppler method depends on the assumption of a flat velocity profile and a constant flow area during the time of the flow. In contrast, the 3D color Doppler quantification of LVOT stroke volume does not require any such assumptions at all. Anyway, when either the 3D color Doppler method or the quantitative 2D method gives the LVOT stroke volume as 62.8 ml and 3D echo shows LVEDV and LVESV to be 200 ml and 120 ml respectively, then MR volume is calculated as

$$3D\ (LVEDV - LVESV) - LVOT\ stroke\ volume = (250 - 140) - 62.8 = 47.2\ ml$$

This value is close enough to the result of the direct PISA method (50 ml). In such a situation, one can be confident about the results of the quantitative analysis. Cross-checking using the 3D LV volume and function method (Figure 6.19), and color 3D or the quantitative PISA method will consolidate the quantitative information about MR volume and overall LV volume and function. I admit that we do not need such calculations or quantification in all the MR patients, but we do need them for certain MR patients such as those with localized wall motion abnormality (LV volume is not obtained that easily by 2D echo) and presumed moderately severe MR. The age of quantitative echocardiography is coming, partly thanks to the development of 3D echocardiography.

CONCLUSION

Three-dimensional echocardiography is indispensable not only for assessment of the morphology of the mitral valve leaflets but also for quantification of the severity of MR.

REFERENCES

1. Spain MG, Smith MD, Grayburn PA Harlamert EA, DeMaria AN. Quantitative assessment of mitral regurgitation by Doppler color flow imaging: angiographic and hemodynamic correlations. J Am Coll Cardiol 1989; 13: 585–90.

2. Helmcke F, Nanda NC, Hsiung MC et al. Color Doppler assessment of mitral regurgitation with orthogonal planes. Circulation 1987; 75: 175–83.

3. Shiota T, Jones M, Teien D et al. Color Doppler regurgitant jet area for evaluating eccentric mitral regurgitation: an animal study with quantified mitral regurgitation. J Am Coll Cardiol 1994; 24: 813–19.

4. Shiota T, Jones M, Teien DE et al. Evaluation of mitral regurgitation using a digitally determined color Doppler flow convergence 'centerline' acceleration method. Studies in an animal model with quantified mitral regurgitation. Circulation 1994; 89: 2879–87.

5. Passafini A, Shiota T, Depp M et al. Factors influencing pulmonary venous flow velocity patterns in mitral regurgitation: an in vitro study. J Am Coll Cardiol 1995; 26: 1333–9.

6. Hall SA, Brickner ME, Willett DL et al. Assessment of mitral regurgitation severity by Doppler color flow mapping of the vena contracta. Circulation 1997; 95: 636–42.

7. Klein AL, Obarski TP, Stewart WJ et al. Transesophageal Doppler echocardiography of pulmonary venous flow: a new marker of mitral regurgitation severity. J Am Coll Cardiol 1991; 18: 518–26.

8. Zhou X, Jones M, Shiota T et al. Vena contracta imaged by Doppler color flow mapping predicts the severity of eccentric mitral regurgitation better than color jet area: a chronic animal study. J Am Coll Cardiol 1997; 30: 1393–8.

9. Tribouilloy C, Shen WF, Quere JP et al. Assessment of severity of mitral regurgitation by measuring regurgitant jet width at its origin with transesophageal Doppler color flow imaging. Circulation 1992; 85: 1248–53.

10. Zoghbi WA, Enriquez-Sarano M, Foster E et al. Recommendations for evaluation of the severity of native valvular regurgitation with two-dimensional and Doppler echocardiography. J Am Soc Echocardiogr 2003; 16: 777–802.

11. Smith MD, Harrison MR, Pinton R et al. Regurgitant jet size by transesophageal compared with transthoracic Doppler color flow imaging. Circulation 1991; 83: 79–86.

12. Hozumi T, Yoshikawa J, Yoshida K et al. Assessment of flail mitral leaflets by dynamic three-dimensional echocardiographic imaging. Am J Cardiol 1997; 79: 223–5.

13. Chauvel C, Bogino E, Clerc P et al. Usefulness of three-dimensional echocardiography for the evaluation of mitral valve prolapse: an intraoperative study. J Heart Valve Dis 2000; 9: 341–9.

14. Delabays A, Jeanrenaud X, Chassot PG, Von Segesser LK, Kappenberger L. Localization and quantification of mitral valve prolapse using three-dimensional echocardiography. Eur J Echocardiogr 2004; 5: 422–9.

15. Macnab A, Jenkins NP, Bridgewater BJ et al. Three-dimensional echocardiography is superior to multiplane transoesophageal echo in the assessment of regurgitant mitral valve morphology. Eur J Echocardiogr 2004; 5: 212–22.

16. Ryan LP, Salgo IS, Gorman RC, Gorman JH 3rd. The emerging role of three-dimensional echocardiography in mitral valve repair. Semin Thorac Cardiovasc Surg 2006; 18: 126–34.

17. Pua EC, Idriss SF, Wolf PD, Smith SW. Real-time 3D transesophageal echocardiography. Ultrason Imaging 2004; 26: 217–32.

18. Handke M, Heinrichs G, Moser U et al. Transesophageal real-time three-dimensional echocardiography methods and initial in vitro and human in vivo studies. J Am Coll Cardiol 2006; 48: 2070–6.

19. Pepi M, Tamborini G, Maltagliati A et al. Head-to-head comparison of two- and three-dimensional transthoracic and transesophageal echocardiography in the localization of mitral valve prolapse. J Am Coll Cardiol 2006; 48: 2524–30.

20. Sugeng L, Coon P, Weinert L et al. Use of real-time 3-dimensional transthoracic echocardiography in the evaluation of mitral valve disease. J Am Soc Echocardiogr 2006; 19: 413–21.

21. De Simone R, Glombitza G, Vahl CF et al. Three-dimensional color Doppler: a clinical study in patients with mitral regurgitation. J Am Coll Cardiol 1999; 33: 1646–54.

22. De Simone R, Glombitza G, Vahl CF et al. Three-dimensional color Doppler: a new approach for quantitative assessment of mitral regurgitant jets. J Am Soc Echocardiogr 1999; 12: 173–85.

23. Li X, Wanitkun S, Li XN et al. Quantification of instantaneous flow rate and dynamically changing effective orifice area using a geometry independent three-dimensional digital color Doppler method: an in vitro study mimicking mitral regurgitation. J Am Soc Echocardiogr 2002; 15: 1189–96.

24. Sitges M, Jones M, Shiota T et al. Real-time three-dimensional color Doppler evaluation of the flow convergence zone for quantification of mitral regurgitation: validation experimental animal study and initial clinical experience. J Am Soc Echocardiogr 2003; 16: 38–45.

25. Mehwald PS, Rusk RA, Mori Y et al. A validation study of aortic stroke volume using dynamic 4-dimensional color Doppler: an in vivo study. J Am Soc Echocardiogr 2002; 15: 1045–50.

26. Li J, Li X, Mori Y et al. Quantification of flow volume with a new digital three-dimensional color Doppler flow approach: an in vitro study. J Ultrasound Med 2001; 20: 1303–11.

27. Tsujino H, Jones M, Qin JX et al. Combination of pulsed-wave Doppler and real-time three-dimensional color Doppler echocardiography for quantifying the stroke volume in the left ventricular outflow tract. Ultrasound Med Biol 2004; 30: 1441–6.

7 Valvular Heart Disease: Mitral Valve; Mitral Annulus and Valve Geometry

Nozomi Watanabe and Kiyoshi Yoshida

Three-dimensional (3D) echocardiography provides a unique en face view of the mitral leaflets and annulus. This technique has been utilized for assessment of the morphologic evaluation of the mitral apparatus in patients with mitral valve disease. However, the quantitative assessment of the mitral apparatus using 3D echocardiography has not been routinely performed because of the cumbersome nature of the measurement procedure. Recent advances in transthoracic real-time echocardiography have finally allowed us to obtain 3D volumetric images easily in the clinical setting. Therefore, a robust method that allows simple 3D quantitative assessment of the mitral apparatus is required.

NOVEL SOFTWARE SYSTEM FOR 3D ANALYSIS OF THE MITRAL APPARATUS

We have developed a new software system, which is designed to visualize 3D images of the whole mitral annulus and leaflets and to analyze them quantitatively using real-time 3D echocardiography.[1] Transthoracic volumetric images that were obtained using full volume mode with the apical view were used for the 3D analysis. Data acquisition was performed by a SONOS 7500® (Philips Ultrasound, Bothell, Washington) ultrasound system with the X4 transducer. All images were digitally stored on compact disk and transferred into a personal computer for off-line analysis. Using our original 3D computer software REAL VIEW® (YD Ltd, Osaka, Japan), the transthoracic 3D volumetric

data (full-volume mode) were automatically cropped into 18 radial planes 10° apart. The mitral annulus and leaflets could be semi-automatically traced. From these data, the anatomic 3D image was reconstructed to demonstrate the actual configuration of the annulus and leaflets with a unique surface coloration where voxels closer to the probe were coded in gradations from blue to red, and this image could be observed from any direction.

QUANTITATIVE ASSESSMENT OF MITRAL VALVE GEOMETRY IN ISCHEMIC MITRAL REGURGITATION

Ischemic mitral regurgitation (MR) has been reported to convey an adverse prognosis after myocardial infarction.[2–4] Though mitral annulus dilatation, tethering of mitral leaflets secondary to left ventricular (LV) dilatation with outward displacement of papillary muscles, and reduced transmitral pressure to coapt the leaflets are implicated as mechanisms for ischemic MR,[5–12] it had been difficult to appreciate the 3D morphology of the complicated mitral valve leaflets and annulus by conventional 2D echocardiography.

Clinical importance of 3D evaluation of mitral geometry in ischemic mitral regurgitation

Ischemic MR is known to occur in patients with systolic LV dysfunction due to ischemic heart disease, with structurally normal mitral valve leaflets.[13]

Clinically important ischemic MR occurs in 20 to 25% of such patients and recent clinical studies have reported that the existence of ischemic MR is associated with excess mortality and risk after myocardial infarction, even after revascularization.[2–4] According to previous experimental and clinical studies, mitral annulus dilatation, tethering of mitral leaflets secondary to LV dilatation (displacement of the attached papillary muscles tethers the mitral leaflets into the LV and restricts their ability to coapt effectively at the level of mitral annulus), and reduced transmitral pressure to coapt the leaflets are implicated as mechanisms for ischemic MR.[6,8–12]

Annuloplasty is currently a common surgical strategy for ischemic/functional MR, even though MR persists after annuloplasty. Recently, new surgical strategies have been anticipated to reduce chronic persistent ischemic MR after annuloplasty. However, in the clinical setting, the degree of geometric change of the mitral leaflets and annulus has previously been assessed in a single slice of the mitral valve component by 2D echocardiography, in spite of the unique configuration of the curved mitral valve and saddle-shaped mitral annulus. Hence, the 2D imaging plane that is currently used for the measurement of tenting length (coaptation length) or tenting area in the clinical studies may miss the maximum tethering site. In addition, present surgical approaches have been developed based on the beneficial results from animal experiments, which do not take into account the variety of 3D geometric deformities in each patient in the clinical setting. A precise and comprehensive understanding of the 3D geometric changes of the whole mitral leaflets and annulus is needed for successful valve repair in the clinical setting.

Geometry of mitral valve apparatus: insights from 3D echocardiography assessment of mitral annular geometry and annular dynamics in ischemic MR

Saddle-shaped non-planarity of the mitral annulus has been previously investigated in animal models using sonomicrometry or marker radiography,[14,15] and in human studies by using hand-rotated 2D or multiplane transesophageal echocardiography.[16,17] This unique characteristic of the mitral annulus configuration is thought to be a more subtle form to optimize mitral leaflet curvature, which minimizes peak mitral leaflet stress[18] and, hence, this curvature might contribute to the mechanisms of avoiding MR, as a part of the 'mitral complex'. Several animal studies have reported the annulus deformation in regional ischemia or in chronic ischemic MR,[15,19] and new surgical strategies to restore the saddle shape of the mitral annulus have been proposed and investigated.[20–22] The saddle shape of the mitral

valve would be much more physiologic and would contribute to successful mitral valve repair in patients with ischemic MR. We demonstrated the curvature of the saddle-shaped mitral annulus in normal subjects. The mitral annulus had its highest points anteriorly near the aortic root and posteriorly near the posterior LV wall, and its low points located in anterior and posterior commissure, as has been reported in previous investigations.[13,16,17]

In patients with infarct LV with LV dysfunction, the saddle shape was deformed to a flat shape, and further deformation was found in patients with ischemic MR.[23] Figure 7.1 shows 3D images of the mitral annulus in a normal subject and in a patient with ischemic MR with LV dysfunction. In the normal subject, the mitral annulus appears as a saddle shape, while in ischemic MR, the annulus is markedly dilated and flattened. We have also reported that the degree of geometric deformation of the annulus was significantly greater in the anterior myocardial infarction group compared with the inferior myocardial infarction group.[24] A recent investigation using 3D echocardiography has shown that the mitral annulus size links LV dilatation to functional MR.[25] There should be geometric heterogeneity in the mitral annulus in ischemic MR associated with variable clinical backgrounds, including the infarct region and infarct size.

Ahmad et al have demonstrated annular motion during the cardiac cycle by using their original computer software system with 3D echocardiography. They found a larger end-diastolic annular perimeter and annular area in ischemic MR patients, with restricted motion in the posterior annulus and increased intertrigonal distance.[26] The same group has also reported that mitral annular motion correlated with left ventricular ejection fraction. The use of 3D echocardiography would contribute to the

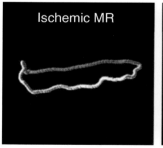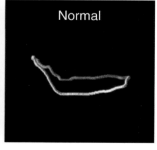

Figure 7.1 Three-dimensional images of the mitral annulus. In a normal subject (right), the mitral annulus appears as a saddle shape, while in ischemic mitral regurgitation, the annulus is dilated and flattened (left). LV, left ventricle; LA, left atrium; A, anterior; P, posterior; M, medial side; L, lateral side.

evaluation of annular dynamics with left atrial/left ventricular function, which has not been well studied.

Assessment of mitral leaflet geometry in ischemic MR

Previous studies have proved that displacement of the attached papillary muscles tethers the mitral leaflets into the LV and restricts their ability to coapt effectively at the level of the mitral annulus, which may also dilate. However, the degree of geometric change of the mitral leaflets and annulus has previously been assessed by 2D echocardiography,[13,27] in spite of the unique configuration of the curved mitral valve and saddle-shaped mitral annulus.[16–19] Kwan et al have reported that the mitral valve tenting in ischemic MR with inferior myocardial infarction was seen asymmetrically in the medial side of the valve by the quantitative measurements performed on selected cut 2D planes obtained from a 3D dataset.[28] We have successfully determined the 3D geometry of the whole mitral leaflets and annulus and quantified the degree of mitral valve tenting and annular deformity in humans by using our original software system. We have clearly shown mitral leaflets globally bulged toward the LV in ischemic MR with global LV dysfunction, clarified the maximum tenting site of the mitral leaflets, and quantified the mitral valve tenting in patients with ischemic MR.[29] Figure 7.2 shows the 3D images of the mitral annulus and leaflets created by Real View®. These 3D images clearly show tethered mitral leaflets in a patient with ischemic MR. In normal subject, leaflets are almost at the level of annulus, which shows a saddle shape. Furthermore, interestingly, in anterior myocardial infarction, mitral valve leaflets were widely tethered toward the LV, in contrast to inferior myocardial infarction which showed localized tenting of the leaflets.[30] Mitral valve geometry in ischemic MR would be heterogeneous in the ischemic MR patients with various types of LV remodeling because of the complicated anatomic and physiologic variability.

Evaluation of geometric changes of the mitral apparatus after surgery

Mitral annuloplasty with reconstructive procedures to restore a more normal alignment between the mitral annulus and displaced papillary muscles is becoming a current surgical strategy for severe ischemic MR.[5] Yamaura et al have investigated mitral annular configuration and dynamics by reconstructed 3D images using transesophageal echocardiography and reported that annular configurations are more physiologic in patients with a flexible annuloplasty ring than in those with a rigid ring.[17,31,32]

However, little is known about the 3D geometric change in the mitral leaflets and annulus after such reconstructive surgery for patients with ischemic MR. We have demonstrated preoperative 3D images showing apparent tenting of the mitral leaflets, which were tethered into the left ventricle. After surgery, the mitral annulus visibly shrank and the mitral leaflet tenting volume was apparently smaller compared with preoperative images (Figure 7.3).[33] Recently, a percutaneous device for mitral regurgitation has been developed and 3D imaging should be the best way to monitor the shape of the mitral leaflets and annulus. Daimon et al have elegantly shown the mitral annular diameter in the anterior–posterior direction after percutaneous mitral valve repair by using real-time 3D echocardiography.[34] A three-dimensional quantitation system would be a unique and helpful tool to evaluate the effects of surgical/non-surgical procedures on the 3D geometry of the mitral apparatus in patients with ischemic MR, and hence to facilitate an informed choice between surgical and non-surgical intervention for each individual.

THREE-DIMENSIONAL EVALUATION OF PAPILLARY MUSCLE POSITION

To understand 3D geometric changes of the mitral apparatus comprehensively, the anatomic position of the papillary muscles in terms of LV geometry should also be evaluated as an important factor in assessing the mechanisms of functional MR. The latest version of our novel software system with transthoracic 3D echocardiography allows us to measure not only tethering lengths but also intrapapillary distance and intrapapillary angle, which can be measured only in 3D datasets. Papillary muscle position changes dynamically along with LV geometry. Figure 7.4 shows the 3D image of the annulus and leaflet with papillary muscle position in a normal subject. In decompensated heart failure with functional MR, mitral valve tenting volume and tenting length decreased with a reduction in annular size with an improvement in heart failure condition. The positions of the papillary muscles shifted after therapy, which should have led to the improvement in mitral tenting and, then, MR volume.[35] Analysis of the dynamics of papillary muscle position should be a key in the process of evaluating the mechanisms of functional MR.

THREE-DIMENSIONAL EVALUATION OF MITRAL GEOMETRY IN MITRAL VALVE PROLAPSE

Accurate determination of a prolapsed leaflet is essential for the successful valve plasty for mitral valve prolapse. Transthoracic and transesophageal

Ischemic MR

Normal

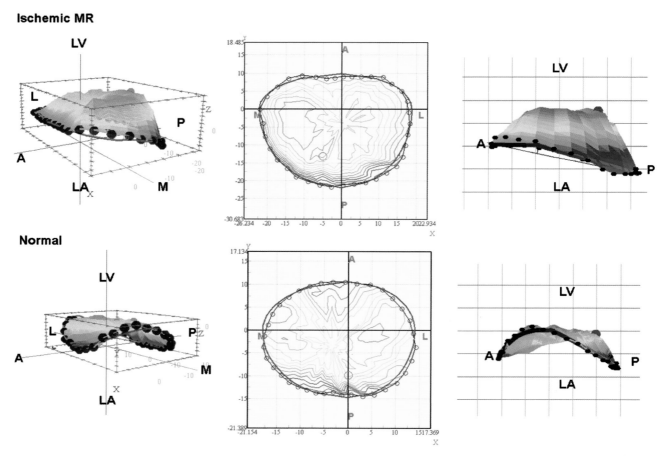

Figure 7.2 Reconstructed 3D images of the mitral leaflets and annulus in ischemic mitral regurgitation (MR) (upper, ischemic MR; lower, normal). In normal subject, leaflets are almost at the level of the annulus, which shows a saddle shape. In a patient with ischemic MR, tethered mitral leaflets and a flattened annulus are clearly seen in the 3D image. LV, left ventricle; LA, left atrium; A, anterior; P, posterior; M, medial side; L, lateral side.

Pre Op

Post Op

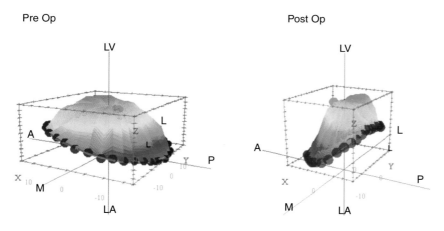

Figure 7.3 Reconstructed 3D images of the mitral leaflets and annulus before and after annuloplastic surgery for ischemic mitral regurgitation. In the preoperative image (left) the mitral annulus is flattened with apparent tenting of the mitral leaflets, showing mountain-shaped leaflet bulging. In the postoperative image (right) the mitral annulus has visibly shrunk and the mitral leaflet tenting volume is apparently smaller. LV, left ventricle; LA, left atrium; A, anterior; P, posterior; M, medial side; L, lateral side.

2D echocardiography is useful in the detection of the prolapsed site.[36,37] Although accuracy in the detection of a prolapsed leaflet is high in 2D studies, it requires appropriate training to achieve an understanding of the unique 3D morphology of a mitral leaflet, which consists of four major scallops (anterior, posterior-medial, middle, and lateral). 3D echocardiography has been anticipated to be a useful diagnostic tool for mitral valve prolapse, and 3D images reconstructed by multiplane transesophageal echocardiography have shown realistic mitral leaflets. The reconstructed, volume-rendered images could be a help in the determination of the prolapsed leaflet site from the left atrium (surgeon's view). However, this technique has not been used in daily clinical practice, since the 3D image construction is time-consuming and the images not suitable for quantitation. By using our newly developed software Real View, we can obtain a 3D image of the prolapsed mitral valve. This image is also available for the quantitation of annular size and degree of prolapse. Figure 7.5 shows the 3D image of the flail leaflet in the posterior middle scallop. We can easily identify the site of prolapse in this image. The depth of the maximum prolapsed site from the level of the mitral annulus was calculated from the 3D dataset to be 16.6 mm in this patient.

FUTURE DIRECTION

To understand 3D geometric changes of the mitral apparatus comprehensively, the anatomic position of the papillary muscles with LV geometry should also be evaluated as an important factor in assessing the mechanisms of functional MR. Analysis of the dynamics of papillary muscle position should be a key in the process of evaluating the mechanism of functional MR. Further clinical trials are needed to evaluate the unique, complex mitral geometry including anatomic and physiologic characteristics and dynamics during the cardiac cycle.

3D evaluation of the mitral valve should be widely applied for mitral valve disease other than ischemic/functional regurgitation. For mitral valve prolapse, which is the most common cause of mitral regurgitation, accurate determination of the prolapsed leaflet is essential for the successful valve plasty for mitral valve prolapse. Although 3D images reconstructed by multiplane transesophageal echocardiography have shown realistic mitral leaflets, this technique has not been used in daily clinical practice since the 3D image construction is time-consuming and the images not suitable for quantitation. Further development of the non-invasive quantitative methods would be a great help for various types of valve disease.

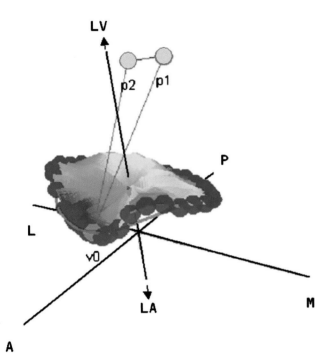

A

Figure 7.4 3D image of the annulus and leaflet with papillary muscle positions. From the 3D datasets, tethering lengths, intrapapillary distance, and intrapapillary angle can be measured. LV, left ventricle; LA, left atrium; A, anterior; P, posterior; M, medial side; L, lateral side; p1, tip of posteromedial papillary muscle; p2, tip of anterolateral papillary muscle.

CONCLUSION

The new quantitative system for 3D echocardiography is a promising technique that can provide precise 3D geometry of the mitral apparatus, which is difficult to elucidate by conventional 2D echocardiography.

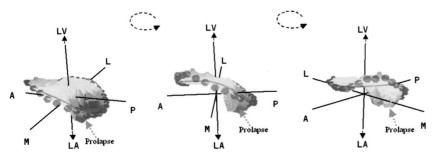

Figure 7.5 3D images of mitral prolapse. Prolapsed leaflet (posterior middle scallop) is clearly identified by reconstructed 3D images. LV, left ventricle; LA, left atrium; A, anterior; P, posterior; M, medial side; L, lateral side.

REFERENCES

1. Yamaura Y, Watanabe N, Ogasawara Y et al. Geometrical demonstration and three-dimensional quantitative analysis of the mitral valve with real time three-dimensional echocardiography: novel anatomical image creation system. J Echocardiogr 2004; 2: 99–104.

2. Tcheng JE, Jackman JD Jr, Nelson CL et al. Outcome of patients sustaining acute ischemic mitral regurgitation during myocardial infarction. Ann Intern Med 1992; 117: 18–24.

3. Lamas GA, Mitchell GF, Flaker GC et al. Clinical significance of mitral regurgitation after acute myocardial infarction. Survival and Ventricular Enlargement Investigators. Circulation 1997; 96: 827–33.

4. Grigioni F, Enriquez-Sarano M, Zehr KJ, Bailey KR, Tajik AJ. Ischemic mitral regurgitation: long-term outcome and prognostic implications with quantitative Doppler assessment. Circulation 2001; 103: 1759–64.

5. Kaul S, Spotnitz WD, Glasheen WP, Touchstone DA. Mechanism of ischemic mitral regurgitation. An experimental evaluation. Circulation 1991; 84: 2167–80.

6. Otsuji Y, Handschumacher MD, Schwammenthal E et al. Insights from three-dimensional echocardiography into the mechanism of functional mitral regurgitation: direct in vivo demonstration of altered leaflet tethering geometry. Circulation 1997; 96: 1999–2008.

7. He S, Fontaine AA, Schwammenthal E, Yoganathan AP, Levine RA. Integrated mechanism for functional mitral regurgitation: leaflet restriction versus coapting force: in vitro studies. Circulation 1997; 96: 1826–34.

8. Messas E, Guerrero JL, Handschumacher MD et al. Paradoxic decrease in ischemic mitral regurgitation with papillary muscle dysfunction: insights from three-dimensional and contrast echocardiography with strain rate measurement. Circulation 2001; 104: 1952–7.

9. Otsuji Y, Handschumacher MD, Liel-Cohen N et al. Mechanism of ischemic mitral regurgitation with segmental left ventricular dysfunction: three-dimensional echocardiographic studies in models of acute and chronic progressive regurgitation. J Am Coll Cardiol 2001; 37: 641–8.

10. Otsuji Y, Kumanohoso T, Yoshifuku S et al. Isolated annular dilation does not usually cause important functional mitral regurgitation: comparison between patients with lone atrial fibrillation and those with idiopathic or ischemic cardiomyopathy. J Am Coll Cardiol 2002; 39: 1651–6.

11. Levine RA, Hung J, Otsuji Y et al. Mechanistic insights into functional mitral regurgitation. Curr Cardiol Rep 2002; 4: 125–9.

12. Lai DT, Tibayan FA, Myrmel T et al. Mechanistic insights into posterior mitral leaflet inter-scallop malcoaptation during acute ischemic mitral regurgitation. Circulation 2002; 106(Suppl): I-40–I-4.

13. Yiu SF, Enriquez-Sarano M, Tribouilloy C, Seward JB, Tajik AJO. Determinants of the degree of functional mitral regurgitation in patients with systolic left ventricular dysfunction: a quantitative clinical study. Circulation 2000; 102: 1400–6.

14. Gorman JH 3rd, Gupta KB, Streicher JT et al. Dynamic three-dimensional imaging of the mitral valve and left ventricle by rapid sonomicrometry array localization. J Thorac Cardiovasc Surg 1996; 112: 712–26.

15. Tibayan FA, Rodriguez F, Langer F et al. Annular remodeling in chronic ischemic mitral regurgitation: ring selection implications. Ann Thorac Surg 2003; 76: 1549–54; discussion 1554–5.

16. Levine RA, Weyman AE, Handschumacher MD. Three-dimensional echocardiography: techniques and applications. Am J Cardiol 1992; 69: 121–30H; discussion 131–4H.

17. Yamaura Y, Yoshikawa J, Yoshida K et al. Three-dimensional analysis of configuration and dynamics in patients with an annuloplasty ring by multiplane transesophageal echocardiography: comparison between flexible and rigid annuloplasty rings. J Heart Valve Dis 1995; 4: 618–22.

18. Salgo IS, Gorman JH 3rd, Gorman RC et al. Effect of annular shape on leaflet curvature in reducing mitral leaflet stress. Circulation 2002; 106: 711–17.

19. Gorman JH 3rd, Jackson BM, Enomoto Y, Gorman RC. The effect of regional ischemia on mitral valve annular saddle shape. Ann Thorac Surg 2004; 77: 544–8.

20. Gillinov AM, Cosgrove DM 3rd, Shiota T et al. Cosgrove–Edwards Annuloplasty System: midterm results. Ann Thorac Surg 2000; 69: 717–21.

21. Gorman JH 3rd, Gorman RC, Jackson BM et al. Annuloplasty ring selection for chronic ischemic mitral regurgitation: lessons from the ovine model. Ann Thorac Surg 2003; 76: 1556–63.

22. Tibayan FA, Rodriguez F, Liang D et al. Paneth suture annuloplasty abolishes acute ischemic mitral regurgitation but preserves annular and leaflet dynamics. Circulation 2003; 108(Suppl 1): II128–33.

23. Watanabe N, Ogasawara Y, Yamaura Y et al. Geometric deformity of the mitral annulus in patients with ischemic mitral regurgitation: a real-time three-dimensional echocardiographic study. J Heart Valve Dis 2005; 14: 447–52.

24. Watanabe N, Ogasawara Y, Yamaura Y et al. Mitral annulus flattens in ischemic mitral regurgitation: geometric differences between inferior and anterior myocardial infarction: a real-time 3-dimensional echocardiographic study. Circulation 2005; 112: I458–62.

25. Popovic ZB, Martin M, Fukamachi K et al. Mitral annulus size links ventricular dilatation to functional mitral regurgitation. J Am Soc Echocardiogr 2005; 18: 959–63.

26. Ahmad RM, Gillinov AM, McCarthy PM et al. Annular geometry and motion in human ischemic mitral regurgitation: novel assessment with three-dimensional echocardiography and computer reconstruction. Ann Thorac Surg 2004; 78: 2063–8; discussion 2068.

27. Kumanohoso T, Otsuji Y, Yoshifuku S et al. Mechanism of higher incidence of ischemic mitral regurgitation in patients with inferior myocardial infarction: quantitative analysis of left ventricular and mitral valve geometry in 103 patients with prior myocardial infarction. J Thorac Cardiovasc Surg 2003; 125: 135–43.

28. Kwan J, Shiota T, Agler DA et al. Geometric differences of the mitral apparatus between ischemic and dilated cardiomyopathy with significant mitral regurgitation: real-time three-dimensional echocardiography study. Circulation 2003; 107: 1135–40.

29. Watanabe N, Ogasawara Y, Yamaura Y et al. Quantitation of mitral valve tenting in ischemic mitral regurgitation by transthoracic real-time three-dimensional echocardiography. J Am Coll Cardiol 2005; 45: 763–9.

30. Watanabe N, Ogasawara Y, Yamaura Y et al. Geometric differences of the mitral valve tenting between anterior and inferior myocardial infarction with significant ischemic mitral regurgitation – quantitation by novel software system with transthoracic real-time three-dimensional echocardiography. J Am Soc Echocardiogr 2006; 19: 71–5.

31. Yamaura Y, Yoshida K, Hozumi T et al. Three-dimensional echocardiographic evaluation of configuration and dynamics of the mitral annulus in patients fitted with an annuloplasty ring. J Heart Valve Dis 1997; 6: 43–7.

32. Yamaura Y, Yoshida K, Hozumi T et al. Evaluation of the mitral annulus by extracted three-dimensional images in patients with an annuloplasty ring. Am J Cardiol 1998; 82: 534–6.

33. Yamaura Y, Watanabe N, Ogasawara Y et al. Geometric change of mitral valve leaflets and annulus after reconstructive surgery for ischemic mitral regurgitation: real-time 3-dimensional echocardiographic study. J Thorac Cardiovasc Surg 2005; 130: 1459–61.

34. Daimon M, Shiota T, Gillinov AM et al. Percutaneous mitral valve repair for chronic ischemic mitral regurgitation: a real-time three-dimensional echocardiographic study in an ovine model. Circulation 2005; 111: 2183–9.

35. Watanabe N, Ogasawara Y, Yamaura Y et al. Dynamics of mitral complex geometry and functional mitral regurgitation during heart failure treatment. J Echocardiogr 2006; 4: 51–8.

36. Yoshida K, Yoshikawa J, Hozumi T et al. Assessment of aortic regurgitation by the acceleration flow signal void proximal to the leaking orifice in cinemagnetic resonance imaging. Circulation 1991; 83: 1951–5.

37. Foster GP, Isselbacher EM, Rose GA et al. Accurate localization of mitral regurgitant defects using multiplane transesophageal echocardiography. Ann Thorac Surg 1998; 65: 1025–31.

8 Valvular Heart Disease: Mitral Valve; Functional Mitral Regurgitation

Jun Kwan

Functional mitral regurgitation (FMR) occurs as a result of cardiomyopathy despite there being a structurally normal mitral valve (MV), and it is a common complication in patients with ischemic heart disease or idiopathic dilated cardiomyopathy (DCM). The tethering of the mitral leaflets caused by a displacement of the papillary muscle (PM) has been thought to be the main mechanism of FMR.[1–6] However, the LV geometry that contributes to a displacement of the PM can vary according to the underlying disease. The LV can be globally remodeled in DCM or locally remodeled in an inferior myocardial infarction (MI). To our knowledge, there are two postero-medial and antero-lateral PMs. Each PM distributes chordae only to the ipsilateral half portion of the MV (Figure 8.1). Therefore, the geometry of the mitral apparatus in FMR, which must be affected by the contributing LV geometry, may be more complicated than previously thought.

With recent advances in real-time 3D echocardiography and 3D computer software, particularly the multiplanar reconstructive (MPR) mode of 3D image analysis, it has become possible to assess the geometry of the cardiac structures with more accuracy than with 2D echocardiography.[7–9]

This chapter discusses the advantages of 3D echocardiography in making geometric measurements of the mitral apparatus in FMR over 2D echocardiography, as well as the geometry of the mitral valve in FMR that is observed with the combined use of 3D echocardiography and the MPR mode of 3D image analysis.

ADVANTAGES OF 3D ECHOCARDIOGRAPHY OVER 2D ECHOCARDIOGRAPHY

Geometry of the mitral valve

Although several new reconstructive surgical procedures to correct FMR have been proposed,[10–12] the surgical treatment is controversial. A better understanding of the MV geometry will help to provide a better rationale for optimal surgical treatment of FMR.

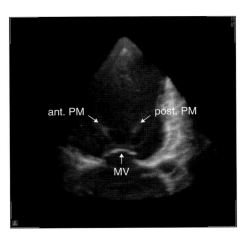

Figure 8.1 3D reconstructed image of LV chamber reveals two papillary muscles (PM) distributing chordae to the ipsilateral half portion of the mitral valve (MV).

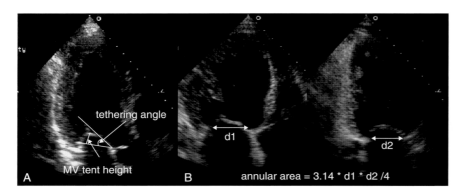

Figure 8.2 Geometric measurement of the mitral valve (MV) using 2D echocardiography. (A) Measurement of the tethering angle and tent height of the MV. (B) Measurement of the dimension and area of the mitral annulus. d1, annular dimension measured on the apical 4-chamber plane; d2, annular dimension measured on the apical 2-chamber plane.

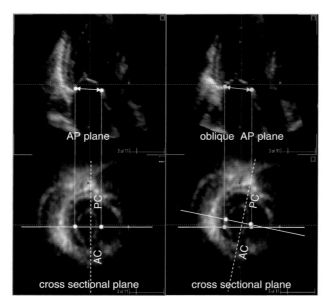

Figure 8.3 Low reproducibility of the annular dimension measurement (white and yellow arrow lines) with 2D echocardiography. Two consecutive apical long axis planes (upper left and right) may neither agree on the cross-sectional plane (lower right) (white and yellow lines) nor cross the identical points of the annulus (lower right) (white and yellow spots). AP, antero-posterior; AC, anterior commissure; PC, posterior commissure.

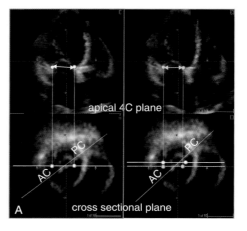

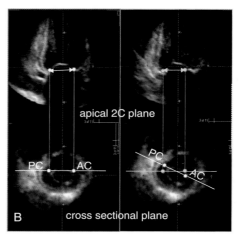

Figure 8.4 Low reproducibility of the annular dimension measurement (white and yellow arrow lines) with 2D echocardiography. (A) Two consecutive apical 4-chamber planes (upper left and right) may neither agree on the cross-sectional plane (lower right) (white and yellow lines) nor cross the identical points of the annulus (lower right) (white and yellow spots). (B) Two consecutive apical 2-chamber planes (upper left and right) may neither agree on the cross-sectional plane (lower right) (white and yellow lines) nor cross the identical points of the annulus (lower right) (white and yellow spots). C, chamber; AC, anterior commissure; PC, posterior commissure.

The geometry of the MV can be assessed by conventional 2D echocardiography, as has been shown in several previous studies[3,13,14] (Figure 8.2). However, accurate information is essential for making geometric measurements of the small cardiac structures such as the annulus or valve, it is, therefore, vital to obtain the same planes that cross identical portions, or intersect at a specific angle, for every measurement in order to ensure the reliability of the measurements. However, this measurement process is not guaranteed when using conventional 2D echocardiography (Figures 8.3 and 8.4) and the consecutive measurements thus have a low reproducibility.

Fortunately, the heart has several well-known anatomic structures that can be used as reference markers. These include the anterior and posterior leaflets, two commissural points, the medial junction

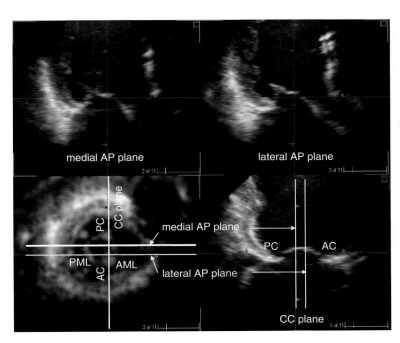

Figure 8.5 Multiplanar reconstructive (MPR) guided acquisition of the medial and lateral antero-posterior (AP) planes. For the anatomic orientation of the mitral annulus (MA), the commissure–commissure (CC) axis connecting the two commissures of the MA is specified in the cross-sectional image at the mitral valve (MV) level and the orthogonal antero-posterior (AP) plane perpendicular to the CC axis is then defined (lower left). By moving the AP plane (white line) from the medial to the lateral side of the MV on the cross-sectional plane (lower left) or CC plane (lower right), 2 AP planes in the medial (upper left) and the lateral (upper right) sides of the MV were obtained. AML, anterior mitral leaflet; PML, posterior mitral leaflet; AC, anterior commissure; PC, posterior commissure.

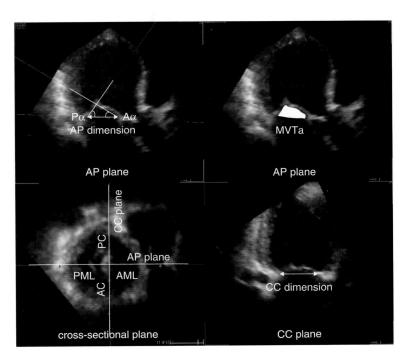

Figure 8.6 Geometric measurement of the mitral valve. Cross-sectional plane of LV at the mitral valve level for the anatomic orientation and the acquisition of the commissure–commissure (CC) and antero-posterior (AP) planes (lower left). The tethering angles of the anterior (Aα) and posterior (Pα) leaflets and the mitral valve area (MVTa) were measured on the AP plane during mid-systole (upper left and right). AP and CC dimensions of the mitral annulus were measured on the AP and CC planes (upper left and lower right). AML, anterior mitral leaflet; PML, posterior mitral leaflet; AC, anterior commissure; PC, posterior commissure.

of the aortic and mitral annuli (MJAM), etc., which are easily delineated in the cross-sectional plane of the LV at the valvular level. This requirement for the accurate delineation of landmarks can be satisfied with the combined use of 3D echocardiography and its cropping method in the MPR mode (Figures 8.5 and 8.6).

The MV geometry can also be assessed three-dimensionally with the appropriate computer software. Watanabe et al[9] reconstructed a 3D image of the MV including the annulus by tracing them in 18 cropped rotational planes using 3D software,

and then successfully demonstrated an MV deformation in ischemic MR.

Geometry of the mitral annulus

Knowledge about the 3D geometry of the mitral annulus (MA) and the changes that occur during the cardiac cycle is very important for understanding the mechanism of FMR in association with the LV geometry. However, the complete structure of the MA and its geometry, which are not visualized on conventional 2D echocardiography, were not

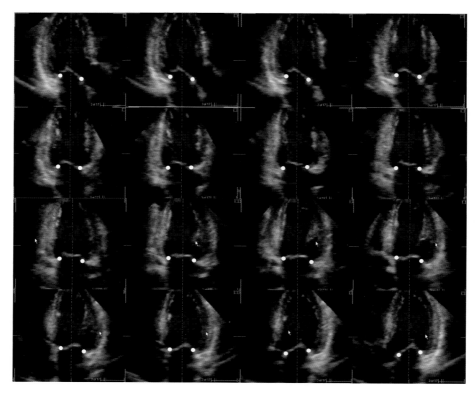

Figure 8.7 Generation of 16 rotational apical planes and tracing of 32 hinge points of the mitral annulus (white spots) for 3D reconstruction of the annulus using newly developed 3D computer software.

clarified until the emergence of 3D echocardiography. Recently, with the advent of 3D computer software, it has become possible to investigate the 3D geometry of the structure with higher accuracy.[9,15–19]

For the reconstruction of the annulus, the LV volumetric data are segmented into multiple rotational apical planes around the long axis of the annulus using 3D software. Two hinge points of the leaflets (the junction points between the annulus and the leaflets) are then traced in each rotational apical plane (Figure 8.7). From these data, the 3D image of the annulus is reconstructed by fitting the images and their interpolation together using 3D computer software.[9,17–19]

For the geometric estimate of the annulus, the coordinate system axes for the anatomic orientation of the MA are then specified in the cross-sectional volumetric images as follows: the commissure–commissure (CC) axis connects the two commissures of the MA; the 2nd orthogonal axis for the MA passes through the intersection of the CC axis in the roughly antero-posterior (AP) direction[16,18,19] (Figure 8.8).

The 2D projected and 3D surface areas of the MA can be automatically calculated from the data fitted by 3D computer software after 3D reconstruction. The non-planarity of the 'saddle-shaped' mitral annulus can be examined by measuring the angle between the anterior and posterior annuli, or the two vectors from the anterior and posterior hinge points of the annulus to the center of the CC axis[16,18,19] (Figures 8.9 and 8.10).

Degree of PM displacement

The PM displacement resulting from the LV wall remodeling is the main underlying geometric cause of the MV tethering in FMR. Therefore, a precise estimation of the degree of PM displacement will provide the critical clue for understanding the heterogeneity of MV tethering in FMR.

Several reports have estimated the PM displacement using 2D echocardiography by measuring the distance between the PM head and certain points.[13,14,20] However, these points are not anatomically defined markers but are defined echocardiographically in certain planes (e.g. parasternal long axis, apical 2- and 4-chamber planes) (Figure 8.11). Therefore, consecutive measurements using this method must have a low reproducibility.

On the other hand, using the MPR guided cropping method, the precise anatomic structures and the anatomic reference points (e.g. PM head, MJAM) can be identified separately. The geometric measurements (e.g. distance or angle) between them will then be completed after placing them on a single plane (Figure 8.12). None of these processes

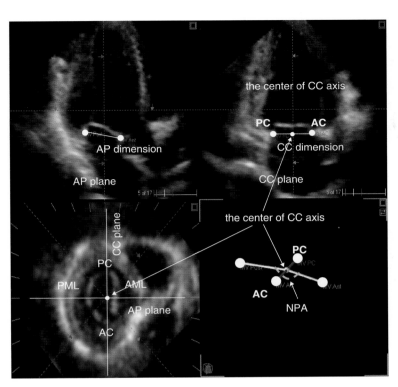

Figure 8.8 Definition of anatomic reference markers of the mitral annulus on the cross-sectional plane and geometric measurements of the annulus. AC, anterior commissure; PC, posterior commissure; AML, anterior mitral leaflet; PML, posterior mitral leaflet; AP, antero-posterior; CC, commissure-commissure; NPA, non-planar angle.

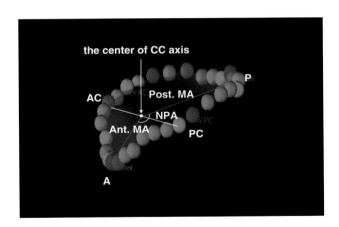

Figure 8.9 Division of the mitral annulus into anterior and posterior annuli by the CC axis and the NPA measurement. CC, commissure–commissure; NPA, non-planar angle, A, anterior point; P, posterior point; AC, anterior commissure; PC, posterior commissure.

are guaranteed when conventional 2D echocardiography is used (Figures 8.13 and 8.14).

Despite the advantages of 3D echocardiography, it still has several disadvantages compared with 2D echocardiography, such as lower temporal and spatial resolution, a narrower angle of image acquisition, and an inability to transfer ECG, etc. Hence, there is a need for significant improvements in both the temporal and spatial resolution in the far field. Moreover, advances in transducer and computer technology are also needed in order

to allow wider angle acquisition and to eliminate the requirement for off-line analysis.

MV DEFORMATION IN FMR

The tethering of both mitral leaflets and their incomplete closure due to the reduced systolic transmitral pressure has been implicated as a main MV deformation in FMR. However, as mentioned earlier, there are two PMs each with chordae distributed only to the ipsilateral half portion of the MV. Therefore, the MV tethering pattern produced by the unilateral PM displacement, which is probably provoked by localized posterior wall remodeling such as lone inferior MI, is expected to be different from the one that occurs with bilateral PM displacement due to global LV remodeling caused by DCM or ischemic cardiomyopathy with chronic severe LV dysfunction.

Heterogeneity of the MV deformation in FMR was first observed by Nielson et al[21] in an in vitro experiment. In that experiment that mimicked the unilateral PM displacement, inconsistent MV tethering was observed. This constituted tethering of both leaflets in the ipsilateral portion of the MV and relative non-tethering of the anterior leaflet, causing prolapse-like deformation in the contralateral portion of the MV to the displaced PM. As suggested in the study, prolapse-like deformation of the contralateral side of the anterior leaflet might develop because this side of the anterior leaflet is

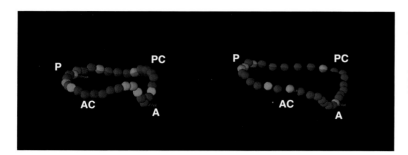

Figure 8.10 Enlarged and flattened mitral annulus in functional mitral regurgitation due to idiopathic dilated cardiomyopathy (right) compared to normal (left). A, anterior point; P, posterior point; AC, anterior commissure; PC, posterior commissure.

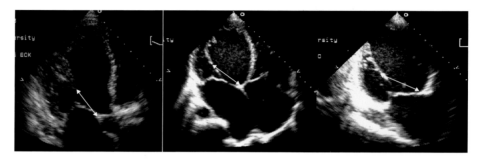

Figure 8.11 Estimation of papillary muscle (PM) displacement using 2D echocardiography. The degree of PM displacement is estimated by measuring the distance (white arrow lines) of the PM head from the anterior annulus on the apical long axis (left), 4-chamber (center), or 2-chamber plane (right).

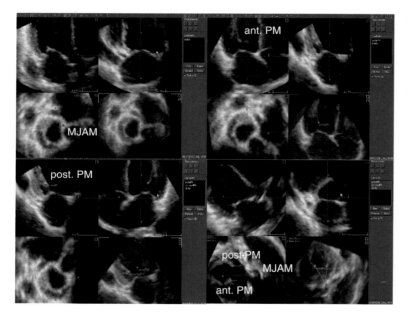

Figure 8.12 Multiplanar reconstructive (MPR) guided measurement of the papillary muscle (PM) displacement. Separate identification is made of the tips of the two PM heads and anatomic reference marker (medial junction between the aortic and mitral annuli [MJAM]) (upper left, upper right, and lower left). Automatic acquisition of the plane displays all structures together for the measurement (lower right).

not tethered and is facing the tethered and restricted posterior leaflet.

The experimental observation of heterogeneity of the MV deformation was demonstrated in a human study with the combined use of 3D echocardiography and the MPR mode of 3D image analysis.[7] In this study, the MV geometry was examined in two FMR patient groups, FMR due to lone inferior MI and FMR due to DCM. The MV deformation was almost consistent in DCM patients, showing tethering of both leaflets from the medial to the lateral side (Figures 8.15 and 8.16). In contrast, it was inconsistent in the inferior MI patients, showing a significant difference in the tethering angle from the medial to the lateral side, particularly the anterior leaflet (Figure 8.17). Consequently, the MV revealed a prolapse-like deformation in the lateral side, as was shown in the previous experimental study.

As the MV deformation in inferior MI differs from that in DCM, the MR jet in the former shows different characteristics (posteriorly directed jet in

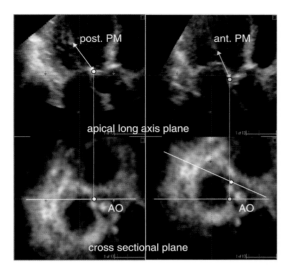

Figure 8.13 Low reproducibility of the PM displacement measurement (white and yellow arrow lines) with 2D echocardiography. Two consecutive apical long axis planes (upper left and right) may neither agree on the cross-sectional plane (lower right) (white and yellow lines) nor cross the identical papillary muscle (PM) head and the identical point of the annulus (lower right) (white and yellow spots). ant. PM, antero-lateral papillary muscle; post. PM, postero-medial papillary muscle; AO, aorta.

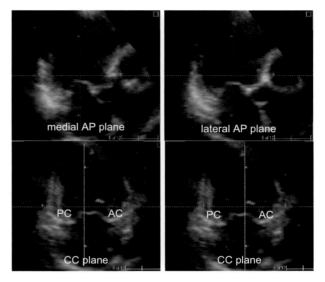

Figure 8.15 Medial (upper left) and lateral (upper right) antero-posterior (AP) planes in functional mitral regurgitation due to idiopathic dilated cardiomyopathy. Both the anterior and posterior leaflets are tethered from the medial to the lateral side during mid-systole. AC, anterior commissure; PC, posterior commissure; CC, commissure–commissure.

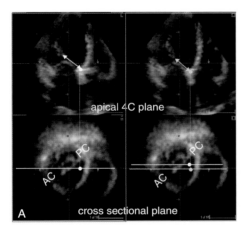

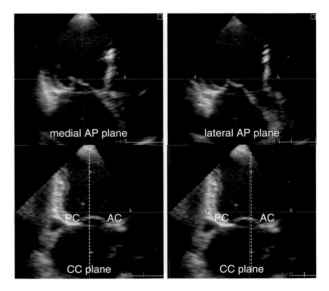

Figure 8.16 Medial (upper left) and lateral (upper right) antero-posterior (AP) planes in functional mitral regurgitation due to ischemic cardiomyopathy with chronic severe LV systolic dysfunction. Both the anterior and posterior leaflets are tethered from the medial to lateral side during mid systole. AC, anterior commissure; PC, posterior commissure; CC: commissure–commissure.

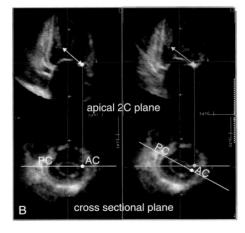

Figure 8.14 Low reproducibility of the PM displacement measurement (white and yellow arrow lines) with 2D echocardiography. (A) Two consecutive apical 4-chamber planes (upper left and right) may neither agree on the

cross-sectional plane (lower right) (white and yellow lines) nor cross the identical point of the annulus (lower right) (white and yellow spots). (B) Two consecutive apical 2-chamber planes (upper left and right) may neither agree on the cross-sectional plane (lower right) (white and yellow lines) nor cross the identical point of the annulus (lower right) (white and yellow spots). AC, anterior commissure; PC, posterior commissure.

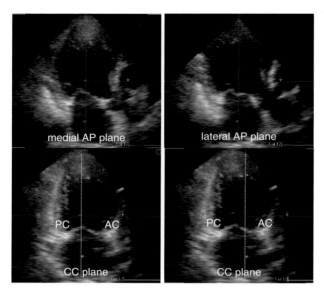

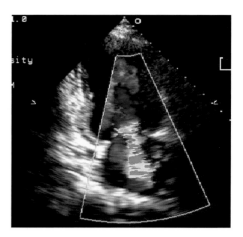

Figure 8.17 Medial (upper left) and lateral (upper right) antero-posterior (AP) planes in functional mitral regurgitation due to lone inferior myocardial infarction. Both the anterior and posterior leaflets are tethered in the medial side, but in the lateral side the anterior leaflet showed preserved motion without tethering during mid-systole. AC, anterior commissure; PC, posterior commissure; CC, commissure–commissure.

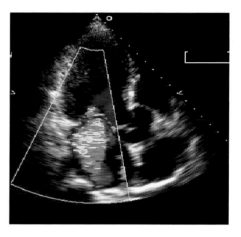

Figure 8.18 Color flow Doppler images showing a wide, single, and centrally directed jet on both apical 2- (left) and 3-chamber (right) planes in dilated cardiomyopathy.

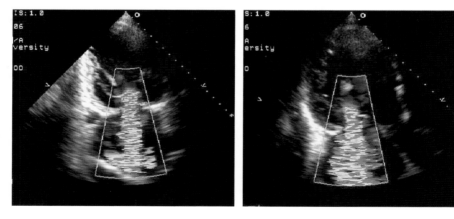

Figure 8.19 Color flow Doppler images showing a wide, single, and centrally directed jet on both apical 2- (left) and 3-chamber (right) planes in ischemic cardiomyopathy with global LV remodeling due to chronic severe LV systolic dysfunction.

the lateral side) from that in the latter (centrally directed jet) (Figures 8.18–8.20).

Recently, Watanabe et al[22] also reported on the geometric differences in the MV deformation between ischemic MR patients due to anterior and inferior MI using 3D echocardiography. In this study, the MV geometry was estimated by reconstructing the 3D shape of the MV using 3D computer software. The MV leaflets were widely tethered toward the LV in an anterior MI, while the MV showed localized tenting in an inferior MI.

These findings suggest that the MV deformation and the geometric mechanisms provoking the consequent MR jet may be different in patients with

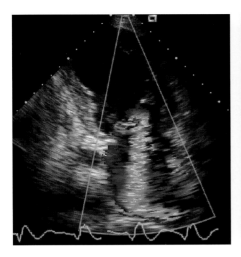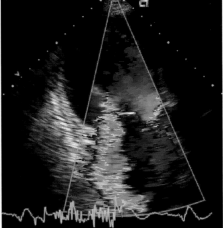

Figure 8.20 Color flow Doppler images showing 2 differently directed jets, one a central jet from the medial portion of the mitral valve, the other a posteriorly directed jet from the lateral portion of the mitral valve on apical 2- (left) and 3-chamber (right) planes in functional mitral regurgitation due to inferior myocardial infarction.

FMR according to the contributing LV geometry (localized or global LV remodeling), which determines the PM displacement (unilateral or bilateral).

CONCLUSION

Several new reconstructive surgical procedures have recently been proposed to correct FMR using animal models.[8–10] However, considering that reconstructive surgery for FMR relies on the morphologic basis of the mitral apparatus, there is a need for better recognition of the geometry of the mitral apparatus. The combined use of 3D echocardiography and the MPR mode for 3D image analysis may provide more detailed information on its geometry than conventional 2D echocardiography and lead to the development of new strategies for the surgical treatment of FMR.

REFERENCES

1. Kaul S, Spotnitz WD, Glasheen WP, Touchstone DA. Mechanism of ischemic mitral regurgitation. An experimental evaluation. Circulation 1991; 84: 2167–80.

2. Kono T, Sabbah HN, Rosman H et al. Mechanism of functional mitral regurgitation during acute myocardial ischemia. J Am Coll Cardiol 1992; 19: 1101–5.

3. Glasson JR, Komeda M, Daughters GT et al. Early systolic mitral leaflet 'loitering' during acute ischemic mitral regurgitation. J Thorac Cardiovasc Surg 1998; 116: 193–205.

4. He S, Fontaine AA, Schwammenthal E, Yoganathan AP, Levine RA. Integrated mechanism for functional mitral regurgitation: leaflet restriction versus coapting force: in vitro studies. Circulation 1997; 96: 1826–34.

5. Otsuji Y, Handschumacher MD, Schwammenthal E et al. Insights from three-dimensional echocardiography into the mechanism of functional mitral regurgitation: direct in vivo demonstration of altered leaflet tethering geometry. Circulation 1997; 96: 1999–2008.

6. Otsuji Y, Handschumacher MD, Liel-Cohen N et al. Mechanism of ischemic mitral regurgitation with segmental left ventricular dysfunction: three-dimensional echocardiographic studies in models of acute and chronic progressive regurgitation. J Am Coll Cardiol 2001; 37: 641–8.

7. Kwan J, Shiota T, Agler DA, et al. Geometric differences of the mitral apparatus between ischemic and dilated cardiomyopathy with significant mitral regurgitation: real-time three-dimensional echocardiography study. Circulation 2003; 107: 1135–40.

8. Song JM, Qin JX, Kongsaerepong V et al. Determinants of ischemic mitral regurgitation in patients with chronic anterior wall myocardial infarction: a real time three-dimensional echocardiography study. Echocardiography 2006; 23: 650–7.

9. Watanabe N, Ogasawara Y, Yamaura Y et al. Quantitation of mitral valve tenting in ischemic mitral regurgitation by transthoracic real-time three-dimensional echocardiography. J Am Coll Cardiol 2005; 45: 763–9.

10. Messas E, Guerrero JL, Handschumacher MD et al. Chordal cutting: a new therapeutic approach for ischemic mitral regurgitation. Circulation 2001; 104: 1958–63.

11. Liel-Cohen N, Guerrero JL, Otsuji Y et al. Design of a new surgical approach for ventricular remodeling to relieve ischemic mitral regurgitation: insights from 3-dimensional echocardiography. Circulation 2000; 101: 2756–63.

12. Mishra YK, Mittal S, Jaguri P, Trehan N. Coapsys mitral annuloplasty for chronic functional ischemic mitral regurgitation: 1-year results. Ann Thorac Surg 2006; 81: 42–6.

13. Yiu SF, Enriquez-Sarano M, Tribouilloy C, Seward JB, Tajik AJ. Determinants of the degree of functional mitral regurgitation in patients with systolic left ventricular dysfunction: a quantitative clinical study. Circulation 2000; 102: 1400–6.

14. Otsuji Y, Kumanohoso T, Yoshifuku S et al. Isolated annular dilation does not usually cause important functional mitral regurgitation: comparison between patients with lone atrial fibrillation and those with idiopathic or ischemic cardiomyopathy. J Am Coll Cardiol 2002; 39: 1651–6.

15. Flachskampf FA, Chandra S, Gaddipatti A et al. Analysis of shape and motion of the mitral annulus in subjects with and without cardiomyopathy by echocardiographic 3-dimensional reconstruction. J Am Soc Echocardiogr 2000; 13: 277–87.

16. Kwan J, Qin JX, Popovic ZB et al. Geometric changes of mitral annulus assessed by real-time 3-dimensional echocardiography: becoming enlarged and less nonplanar in the anteroposterior direction during systole in proportion to global left ventricular systolic function. J Am Soc Echocardiogr 2004; 17: 1179–84.

17. Watanabe N, Ogasawara Y, Yamaura Y et al. Mitral annulus flattens in ischemic mitral regurgitation: geometric differences between inferior and anterior myocardial infarction: a real-time 3-dimensional echocardiographic study. Circulation 2005; 112: I458–62.

18. Nii M, Roman KS, Macgowan CK, Smallhorn JF. Insight into normal mitral and tricuspid annular dynamics in pediatrics: a real-time three-dimensional echocardiographic study. J Am Soc Echocardiogr 2005; 18: 805–14.

19. Kwan J, Kim G, Jeon M et al. 3D geometry of a normal tricuspid annulus during systole; a comparison study with the mitral annulus using real-time 3D echocardiography. Eur J Echocardiogr 2007.

20. Kumanohoso T, Otsuji Y, Yoshifuku S et al. Mechanism of higher incidence of ischemic mitral regurgitation in patients with inferior myocardial infarction: quantitative analysis of left ventricular and mitral valve geometry in 103 patients with prior myocardial infarction. J Thorac Cardiovasc Surg 2003; 125: 135–43.

21. Nielsen SL, Nygaard H, Fontaine AA et al. Papillary muscle misalignment causes multiple mitral regurgitant jets: an ambiguous mechanism for functional mitral regurgitation. J Heart Valve Dis 1999; 8: 551–64.

22. Watanabe N, Ogasawara Y, Yamaura Y et al. Geometric differences of the mitral valve tenting between anterior and inferior myocardial infarction with significant ischemic mitral regurgitation: quantitation by novel software system with transthoracic real-time three-dimensional echocardiography. J Am Soc Echocardiogr 2006; 19: 71–5.

9 Valvular Heart Disease: Mitral Valve; Mitral Stenosis

Takahiro Shiota

CLINICAL TWO-DIMENSIONAL ECHOCARDIOGRAPHY

Mitral stenosis (MS) is caused by rheumatic valve disease in most patients (Figure 9.1), while occasionally, congenital parachute mitral valve (Figure 9.2), radiation, extensive annular calcification, bacterial endocarditis (vegetation), and myxoma may be the hemodynamic cause of mitral stenosis. Conventional two-dimensional (2D) echocardiography demonstrates such anatomic abnormalities, including leaflet mobility, leaflet thickness, leaflet calcification, and subvalvular and commissural fusion. Severity of MS is also determined by conventional 2D echocardiography. Normal mitral valve area (MVA) is considered to be more than 4 cm^2; MVA $\leq$ 1.0 cm^2 is considered to be severe MS; 1.0 cm^2 < MVA $\leq$ 1.5 cm^2, moderate MS; and 1.5 cm^2 < MVA $\leq$ 2.0 cm^2, mild MS. There are quite a few echocardiographic methods for determining the severity of MS, including 2D planimetry, continuous wave (CW) Doppler pressure half time, and the proximal isovelocity surface area (PISA) or flow convergence (FC) method.[1–9] MVA should be determined by using all available methods and cross-checking the values in patients with MS.

Two-dimensional planimetry method (Figure 9.3)

Many echocardiographic methods for evaluating the severity of MS have been proposed and published in a variety of cardiology and ultrasound journals. Among them, 2D planimetry is probably one of the most widely used methods for judging the severity of MS (Figure 9.3).[1–3,9] When one attempts to measure the mitral valve area by this method, it is imperative to obtain the real parasternal short-axis view of the mitral valve with proper gain settings and measure the smallest area by tracing the tip of the mitral leaflets. Oblique short-axis 2D views

may result in overestimation of the actual mitral valve area while overgain imaging of severely calcified valves may underestimate the real area. Three-dimensional (3D) echocardiography may be able to overcome this often vital shortcoming of the current 2D echo by rotating perspective views of the mitral valve. However, one must be careful about the thickness of the leaflet when 3D echo is applied to determine MV area because of the thicker presentation of the mitral valve leaflets expected by this new method.

Pressure half time method (Figure 9.4)

Impedance against the transmitral flow during diastole results in a filling prolongation, which is a

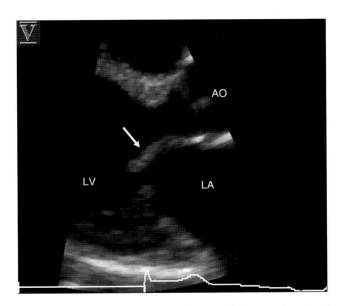

Figure 9.1 Typical parasternal view of rheumatic mitral stenosis. Doming of the anterior leaflet (arrow) is the hallmark of rheumatic valve disease and is well recognized in this 2D view. However, this 2D image cannot show how wide the doming is from the lateral to medial side. AO, aorta; LA, left atrium; LV, left ventricle.

longer duration of the pressure drop from the beginning to half of the pressure gradient (pressure half time, PHT) in patients with MS.[4,5] Empirically, MVA is determined by the following equation:

$$MVA \ (cm^2) = 220/PHT \ (m \ s)$$

When aortic regurgitation (AR) coexists with mitral stenosis, this method would overestimate the MVA because AR causes the rapid pressure rise of the left ventricle during diastole, resulting in shorter PHT.[10] The CW Doppler method provides another important piece of information in patients with MS: the peak and mean pressure gradient between LV and LA. In particular, the mean pressure gradient obtained by tracing the CW envelope provides an estimate of the severity of MS (Figure 9.5). A mean pressure gradient < 12 mmHg suggests severe MS, 5 mmHg ≤ mean pressure gradient < 12 mmHg, moderate MS, and mean pressure gradient < 5 mmHg, mild MS.

The increased left atrial pressure caused by MS eventually results in pulmonary hypertension in patients with MS. Pulmonary artery systolic pressure is also estimated by conventional echocardiography using the simplified Bernoulli equation; the

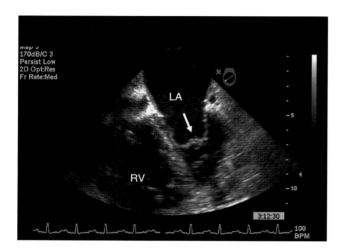

Figure 9.2   Congenital mitral stenosis. An example of a 2D transesophageal echocardiography image, demonstrating a congenital parachute mitral valve (arrow), causing hemodynamically severe mitral stenosis. LA, left atrium; RV, right ventricle.

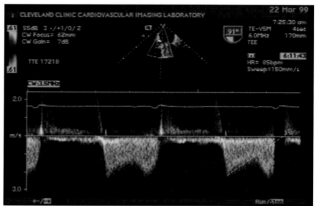

PHT = 167 ms

Figure 9.4   A CW Doppler recording of transmitral flow in a patient with mitral stenosis. Pressure half time (PHT) is measured from the deceleration slope. Mitral valve area is determined by the equation, 220/PHT. In this case, MVA was 220/167, 1.3 cm². However, no one can be sure that the CW curser line is placed on the exact direction of the transmitral inflow.

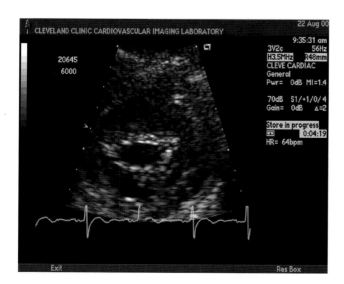

Figure 9.3   A parasternal short-axis view of the mitral valve. By tracing the tip of the leaflets, one can determine mitral valve area. No one can be sure, however, that this is the smallest valve area by using only 2D echocardiography.

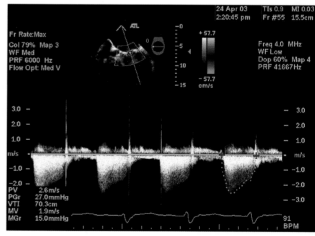

Figure 9.5   A CW Doppler recording from a patient with severe MS. After tracing the envelope of the velocity, the mean pressure gradient was found to be 15 mmHg.

pressure gradient between RA and RV $= 4V_{max}^2$, where Vmax (m/s) is the maximal velocity of tricuspid regurgitation (Figures 9.6 and 9.7).[4] Thus, when we assume RA pressure to be 5 mmHg, RV systolic and PA systolic pressure (in the absence of pulmonary stenosis) $= 4V_{max}^2 + 5$.

When one attempts to measure the mitral valve area and PA pressure by the CW method, it is imperative to place the CW Doppler interrogation line parallel to the direction of the blood flow. However, conventional 2D echo may not provide accurate spatial information about the exact location of the CW interrogation line relative to the blood flow, resulting in erroneous or uncertain estimation of the valve area and pressure. 3D echocardiography can guide the precise placement of the CW Doppler

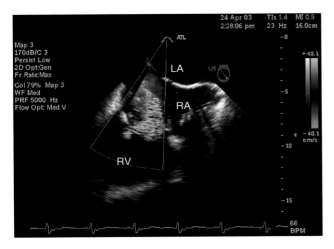

Figure 9.6 An example of a 2D TEE image in a patient with severe MS, demonstrating moderate tricuspid regurgitation. LA, left atrium; RA, right atrium; RV, right ventricle.

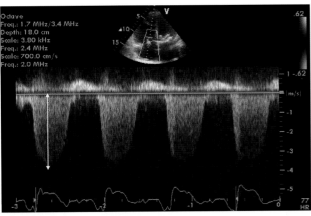

Peak velocity of 3.6 m/sec

Figure 9.7 An example of CW Doppler recording of tricuspid regurgitation from a patient with severe MS and pulmonary hypertension. Systolic pulmonary artery pressure was estimated as 57 mmHg by employing the simplified Bernoulli equation. However, again, no one can be sure that the CW curser line is placed on the exact direction of the TR jet.

interrogation line to further improve the accuracy of this CW method.

Flow convergence method or PISA method (Figure 9.8)

Color Doppler imaged flow convergence towards the stenotic mitral valve (or PISA) can provide an alternative technique for determining MVA.[7,8] In this method, assuming a hemispheric shape of PISA, MVA is derived from the following equation:[7]

$$MVA = 2 \times \pi \times R^2 \times Vn/Vmax$$

where Vn = Nyquist velocity and Vmax = CW maximal velocity of transmitral inflow. However, when the inlet angle (θ°) is significant, it is necessary to use a correction factor as follows:[7]

$$MVA \text{ corrected} = MVA \times \theta°/180°$$

3D echocardiography should improve this method by demonstrating a more realistic shape of PISA, which is not a hemisphere in MS, as will be discussed later.

BALLOON MITRAL VALVULOPLASTY

Balloon mitral valvuloplasty or commissurotomy is indicated in symptomatic patients (New York Heart Association functional class (NYHA class 2 ≤)) with moderate or severe MS (MVA ≤ 1.5 cm²) and a valve morphology favorable for this procedure with an absence of LA thrombus or moderate to severe MR.[11,12] Asymptomatic patients with

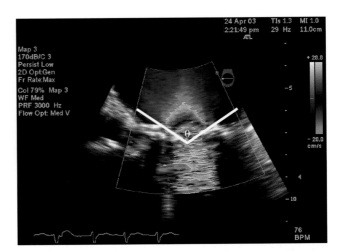

Figure 9.8 An example of PISA or flow convergence towards a stenotic mitral valve. The mitral valve is determined by an angle-corrected PISA method (see text).

MVA $\leq$ 1.5 cm^2 and pulmonary hypertension (pulmonary artery systolic pressure < 50 mmHg at rest or < 60 mmHg at peak exercise) may be considered for this procedure.

Conventional 2D echocardiography plays a key role to provide valve morphology, the degree of stenosis and regurgitation, and pulmonary artery systolic pressure. Echocardiographic score of the morphologic abnormality of the mitral valve apparatus is widely used for determining suitability of valvuloplasty, and a total score of 8 or less is considered to be a favorable morphology for this procedure.[11,12] However, in actual clinical settings, one must not apply this echocardiographic score rigidly, particularly in intermediate cases because there exists significant overlap of the outcome in these patients and uncertainty of the scoring itself, with relatively high observer variability.[12]

When the procedure is executed, real-time 3D echo as well as conventional 2D echo, including TEE, can provide vital information on the location of the catheter and balloon, and changes in the severity of MS and MR during this procedure.

APPLICATION OF 3D ECHOCARDIOGRAPHY

What is the additional value of 3D echocardiography for assessing mitral stenosis? First, the geometry of the mitral valve can be demonstrated by 3D echocardiography, as seen in Figure 9.9. Second, as mentioned above, the stenotic valve area can be determined by using unique 3D views.

Different 3D echo methods were used to determine the valve area in patients with mitral stenosis.[13–17] Binder et al. reported real-time volumetric 3D echo data for the estimation of mitral valve area in patients with mitral valve stenosis.[14] In 48 patients with mitral stenosis, MVA was determined by planimetry using volumetric real-time 3D echo and compared to measurements obtained by 2D echo and Doppler pressure half time (PHT). While 2D echo allowed planimetry of the mitral valve in 43 of 48 patients (89%), calculation of the MVA was possible in all patients when 3D echo was used. Mitral valve area by 3D echo correlated well with MVA by 2D echo ($r = 0.93$, mean difference, 0.09 cm^2) and by PHT ($r = 0.87$, mean difference, 0.16 cm^2). Interobserver variability was significantly less for 3D echo than for 2D echo (SD 0.08 cm^2 versus SD 0.23 cm^2, $p < 0.001$).

In this study, 3D echo reportedly provided accurate and highly reproducible measurements of mitral valve area and can easily be performed from an apical approach. In another study, a more recent type of real-time 3D echo system was used for planimetry. This was reportedly more accurate than the Gorlin method to measure the valve area although the authors used three classical 2D echo methods (2D planimetry, pressure half time, and the PISA method) as the reference method. The authors concluded in this study that we should keep in mind that 3D echo planimetry may be a better reference method than the Gorlin method to assess the severity of rheumatic mitral stenosis.[16]

When 2D methods are used as reference, one may wonder whether 3D echocardiography can be used independently or not in the clinical setting. I personally believe that the combination of conventional 2D echo especially with CW Doppler (for determining pressure gradients and pressure half time) and 3D echo is the best way to accurately assess pathophysiology and hemodynamics in patients with MS. As we all know, one should use multiple echo methods to cross-check the values (MVA and pressure gradients), whether those are 2D or 3D methods.

The most striking information by 3D echocardiography is the depth and spatial relationship between

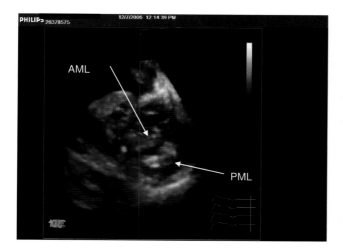
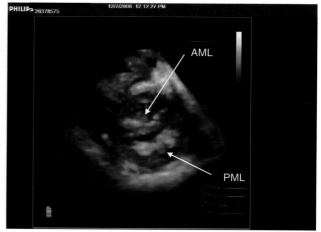

Figure 9.9 Two different views of a stenotic mitral valve by 3D echocardiography. Note that a severe stenosis is well recognized in these 3D views. AML, anterior mitral leaflet; PML, posterior mitral leaflet.

two leaflets revealed by rotation of the mitral valve image in motion (Figures 9.9–9.12). Not only the severity of the stenosis but also the shape, location, and anatomic abnormalities of the mitral valve leaflets such as heavy calcification are visualized in a most intuitive way. Also, 3D PISA images give us clear insight for the location and shape of PISA in MS. As stated before, the 2D PISA method assumes a hemispheric shape of PISA to determine MVA, whether the angle is corrected or not. However, as seen in Figure 9.13 (right panel), the shape of PISA showed an elongated, crescent shape of non-hemispheric geometry. This indicates the absolute necessity of an appropriate correction to use the simple PISA method for determining the MV area with high accuracy.

APPLICATION OF 3D ON BALLOON MITRAL VALVULOPLASTY

Application of 3D echocardiography for valvuloplasty has been reported many times.[18,19] In one of these studies, multiplane transesophageal echocardiography (TEE with electrocardiographic and respiratory cycle gated image acquisition) was used in 19 patients undergoing balloon mitral valvuloplasty. The mitral valve was viewed *en face* as if looking up from the left ventricle. The mean mitral valve area (by pressure half time from the Doppler of the 2D echocardiogram) increased after valvuloplasty from 0.86 ± 0.06 cm^2 to 2.07 ± 0.10 cm^2, $p < 0.0001$. This was similar to the mitral valve areas obtained by planimetry from 3D images.

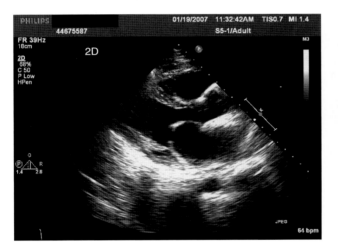
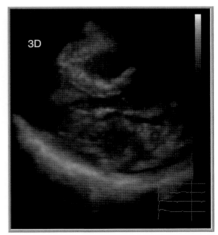

Figure 9.10 Direct comparison of 2D and 3D parasternal views from the same patient with rheumatic mitral stenosis. In the 2D view (left), connections between the leaflets and chords are not recognized as well as in the 3D view (right).

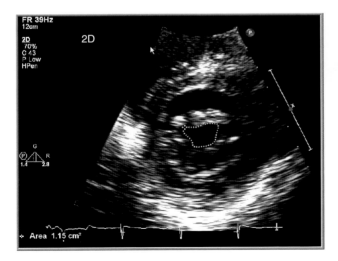
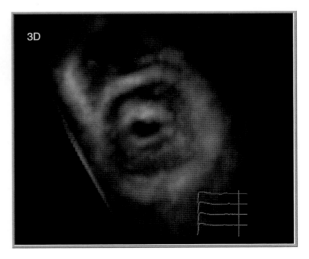

Figure 9.11 Direct comparison of 2D and 3D short-axis views from the same patient with rheumatic mitral stenosis. In the 2D view (left), only a part of both anterior and posterior leaflets is visualized while the entire valve is visualized with the smallest stenotic orifice in the 3D view (right).

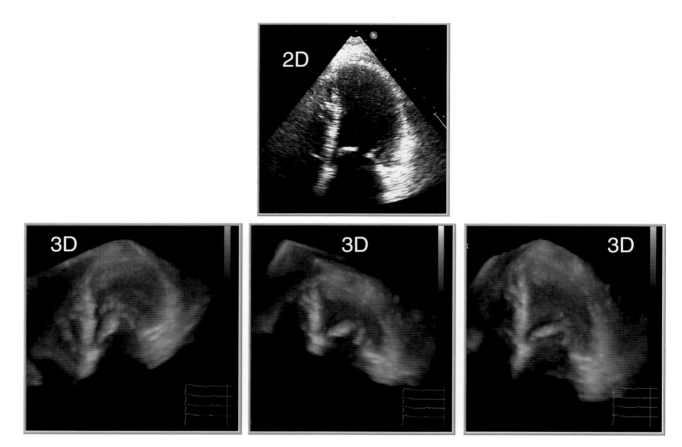

Figure 9.12 Direct comparison of 2D and 3D apical views from the same patient with rheumatic mitral stenosis. In the 2D view (above), doming of the anterior leaflet is seen as a curved line while in 3D views, the doming is seen as a curved plane (below).

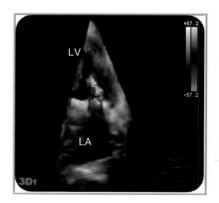 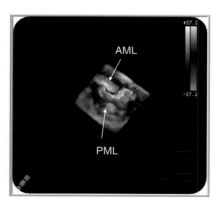

Figure 9.13 3D PISA in MS. PISA is seen in the vertical or apical (left) and horizontal (right) views. PISA shape is completely different between these two views. Note that the left panel is a view from the left atrium, and thus color coding is opposite to the right panel. LA, left atrium; LV, left ventricle; AML, anterior mitral leaflet; PML, posterior mitral leaflet.

3D reconstructions showed a complete commissural split in 10 patients and partial splitting in 9 patients. In 3 of the 8 patients who had an increase in the amount of mitral regurgitation, 3D reconstructions were able to detect tears within the valve leaflet. One leaflet tear actually extended up to the mitral valve annulus and was associated with the only case of severe mitral regurgitation. The authors then concluded that 3D echocardiographic reconstruction enabled visualization of the mitral valve so that commissural splitting and leaflet tears not seen on 2D echocardiography became visible.[18]

Thanks to recent developments in relatively high-quality transthoracic real-time 3D echocardiography, improvement in measurement of valve area and changes in valve geometry after the balloon valvuloplasty was reported.[19] Transthoracic real-time 3D echo, instead of multiplane TEE 3D reconstruction, could be employed to measure the valve area in 29 patients with rheumatic mitral stenosis who underwent balloon valvuloplasty.[19] The authors also concluded that transthoracic real-time 3D echo was a feasible and accurate technique for measuring mitral valve area in patients with rheumatic mitral valve stenosis.

Color 3D images may enhance our understanding of the increase in mitral inflow and changes in the shape of the orifice after the procedure through the location and geometry of the PISA. In view of the new development of transesophageal real-time 3D echocardiography, it may be possible to monitor the procedure in real time in the catheterization laboratory in the near future.

CONCLUSION

The newly developed real-time 3D echocardiography with color Doppler capability not only demonstrates realistic views of the entire stenotic mitral valve, but also the shape of flow convergence (PISA) toward the stenotic valve. Percutaneous balloon valvuloplasty will be better monitored by TEE-based real-time 3D echocardiography than by conventional 2D echocardiographic methods.

REFERENCES

1. Henry WL, Griffith JM, Michaelis LL et al. Measurement of mitral orifice area in patients with mitral valve disease by real-time, two-dimensional echocardiography. Circulation 1975; 51: 827–31.

2. Nichol PM, Gilbert BW, Kisslo JA. Two-dimensional echocardiographic assessment of mitral stenosis. Circulation 1977; 55: 120–8.

3. Wann LS, Weyman AE, Feigenbaum H et al. Determination of mitral valve area by cross-sectional echocardiography. Ann Intern Med 1978; 88: 337–41.

4. Brubakk AO, Angelsen BA, Hatle L. Diagnosis of valvular heart disease using transcutaneous Doppler ultrasound. Cardiovasc Res 1977; 11: 461–9.

5. Hatle L, Brubakk A, Tromsdal A et al. Noninvasive assessment of pressure drop in mitral stenosis by Doppler ultrasound. Br Heart J 1978; 40: 131–40.

6. Nakatani S, Masuyama T, Kodama K et al. Value and limitations of Doppler echocardiography in the quantification of stenotic mitral valve area: comparison of the pressure half-time and the continuity equation methods. Circulation 1988; 77: 78–85.

7. Rodriguez L, Thomas JD, Monterroso V et al. Validation of the proximal flow convergence method. Calculation of orifice area in patients with mitral stenosis. Circulation 1993; 88: 1157–65.

8. Shiota T, Jones M, Valdes-Cruz LM et al. Color flow Doppler determination of transmitral flow and orifice area in mitral stenosis: experimental evaluation of the proximal flow-convergence method. Am Heart J 1995; 129: 114–23.

9. Faletra F, Pezzano A Jr, Fusco R et al. Measurement of mitral valve area in mitral stenosis: four echocardiographic methods compared with direct measurement of anatomic orifices. J Am Coll Cardiol 1996; 28: 1190–7.

10. Flachskampf FA, Weyman AE, Gillam L et al. Aortic regurgitation shortens Doppler pressure half-time in mitral stenosis: clinical evidence, in vitro simulation and theoretic analysis. J Am Coll Cardiol 1990; 16: 396–404.

11. Wilkins GT, Weyman AE, Abascal VM, Block PC, Palacios IF. Percutaneous balloon dilatation of the mitral valve: an analysis of echocardiographic variables related to outcome and the mechanism of dilatation. Br Heart J 1988; 60: 299–308.

12. Abascal VM, Wilkins GT, O'Shea JP et al. Prediction of successful outcome in 130 patients undergoing percutaneous balloon mitral valvotomy. Circulation 1990; 82: 448–56.

13. Chen Q, Nosir YF, Vletter WB et al. Accurate assessment of mitral valve area in patients with mitral stenosis by three-dimensional echocardiography. J Am Soc Echocardiogr 1997; 10: 133–40.

14. Binder TM, Rosenhek R, Porenta G, Maurer G, Baumgartner H. Improved assessment of mitral valve stenosis by volumetric real-time three-dimensional echocardiography. J Am Coll Cardiol 2000; 36: 1355–61.

15. Sugeng L, Weinert L, Lammertin G et al. Accuracy of mitral valve area measurements using transthoracic rapid freehand 3-dimensional scanning: comparison with noninvasive and invasive methods. J Am Soc Echocardiogr 2003; 16: 1292–300.

16. Perez de Isla L, Casanova C, Almeria C et al. Which method should be the reference method to evaluate the severity of rheumatic mitral stenosis? Gorlin's method versus 3D-echo. Eur J Echocardiogr 2006; (in press)

17. Sugeng L, Coon P, Weinert L et al. Use of real-time 3-dimensional transthoracic echocardiography in the evaluation of mitral valve disease. J Am Soc Echocardiogr 2006; 19: 413–21.

18. Applebaum RM, Kasliwal RR, Kanojia A et al. Utility of three-dimensional echocardiography during balloon mitral valvuloplasty. J Am Coll Cardiol 1998; 32: 1405–9.

19. Zamorano J, Perez de Isla L, Sugeng L et al. Non-invasive assessment of mitral valve area during percutaneous balloon mitral valvuloplasty: role of real-time 3D echocardiography. Eur Heart J 2004; 25: 2086–91.

10 Valvular Heart Disease: Aortic Valve

Nozomi Watanabe and Kiyoshi Yoshida

Two-dimensional (2D) echocardiography is limited with the need of geometric assumption in the assessment of valve geometry and in the quantification of regurgitation. Transesophageal three-dimensional (3D) echocardiography has been developed and the usefulness of this new imaging technique in the assessment of the aortic valve has been reported.[1] Transthoracic 3D echocardiograpy is now available, which provides a simple means to scan the whole heart non-invasively. Transthoracic real-time color Doppler 3D echocardiography can capture the entire flow signal, providing unique information on its shape and location, and permitting reliable quantification of aortic regurgitation.[2]

BIPLANE AND FULL-VOLUME THREE-DIMENSIONAL ECHOCARDIOGRAPHY

Full-volume 3D echocardiography can provide a pyramidal image of the whole heart and the volume-rendered image can be rotated and observed from any direction. Although the image quality of current real-time 3D echocardiography is lower than conventional 2D echocardiography, full-volume 3D images help the observer to understand the exact anatomic position of each structure. The aortic valve can be observed from the direction of the ascending aorta, which is impossible by 2D echocardiography. Figure 10.1(A) shows the bicuspid aortic valve by 2D and full-volume 3D echocardiography. In the 3D view, the bicuspid valve is clearly seen from inside the ascending aorta.

By utilizing biplane 3D echocardiography, a heart can be visualized from two different views simultaneously. The degree of the cutting planes and cropping axis can be freely changed. The biplane 3D image helps us to understand the exact position of the probe, and by looking at these images simultaneously in real time, the 3D configuration of the heart structure can be easily understood. Figure 10.1(B) shows the images of the bicuspid aortic valve produced by biplane 3D echocardiography. In this mode, the bileaflet aortic valve with leaflet doming can be clearly visualized, in long-axis and short-axis views of the aortic valve. The cropping axis is set across the aortic valve in this view. 3D echocardiography can give us more accurate anatomic information than conventional 2D echocardiography. Poutanen et al measured the aortic valve annulus areas in 168 healthy children and young adults by 3D echocardiography and found that the aortic annular area increases linearly in relation to body size.[3]

Three-dimensional observation of the aortic valve provides unique additional information in the diagnosis of various types of aortic valve disease. Miyamoto et al reported a case with discrete subaortic stenosis diagnosed by 2D and 3D echocardiography. In this unusual case with complicated morphology, 3D echocardiography provided useful anatomic and functional information, which was helpful before surgical intervention.[4]

THREE-DIMENSIONAL COLOR DOPPLER ECHOCARDIOGRAPHY

3D color Doppler facilitates morphologic assessment of the flow jet and helps to appreciate the 3D vena contracta with acceleration flow. The regurgitant orifice is often an elliptic or irregular oval, which

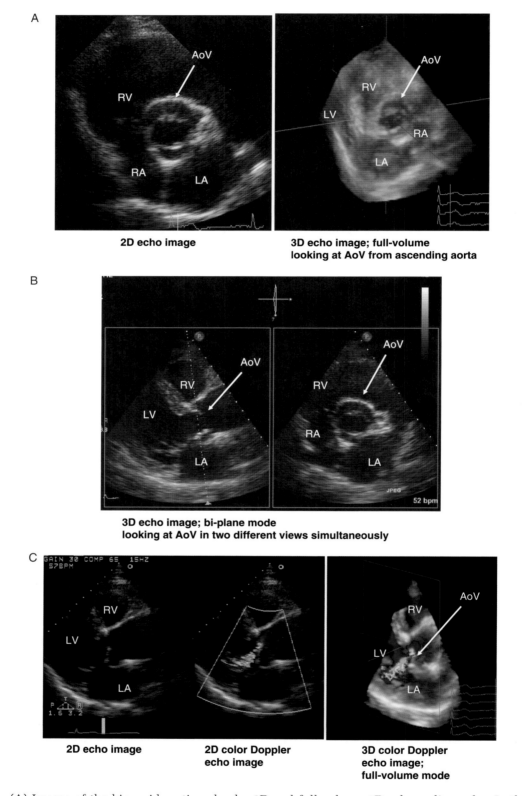

A

2D echo image   3D echo image; full-volume
                             looking at AoV from ascending aorta

B

3D echo image; bi-plane mode
looking at AoV in two different views simultaneously

C

2D echo image   2D color Doppler   3D color Doppler
                     echo image   echo image;
                                             full-volume mode

Figure 10.1 (A) Images of the bicuspid aortic valve by 2D and full-volume 3D echocardiography. In the 3D view, the bicuspid valve is clearly seen from inside the ascending aorta. The pyramidal image from the parasternal approach is cropped from the direction of the ascending aorta. (B) Images of the bicuspid aortic valve by biplane 3D echocardiography. The bileaflet aortic valve with leaflet doming can be clearly visualized simultaneously in the parasternal long-axis and short-axis views of the aortic valve. The cropping axis is set across the aortic valve. (C) 2D and 3D color Doppler image clearly shows regurgitant orifice (arrow). LV, left ventricle; LA, left atrium; RV, right ventricle; RA, right atrium; AOV; aortic valve.

changes the width of the vena contracta in different views. 3D color Doppler echocardiography is a useful tool in the visualization of the actual shape of the regurgitant orifice.[5,6] In other words, the 3D echocardiographic image allows us to measure the vena contracta area. Fung et al investigated the accuracy of the vena contracta area measurements by live 3D color Doppler echo cardiography in aortic regurgitation.[6]

Figure 10.2 shows a case of aortic regurgitation. In 2D echocardiography, moderate regurgitation with irregular proximal isovelocity surface area (PISA) is seen. 3D color Doppler echocardiography shows that this patient actually has two regurgitant orifices. When the gray-scale image is suppressed

to view the regurgitant jet, two regurgitant orifices are more clearly seen and by rotating the image from inside the ascending aorta, two flow jets are observed passing through the aortic valve.

PITFALLS IN THE ASSESSMENT OF THE AORTIC VALVE BY REAL-TIME 3D ECHOCARDIOGRAPHY

3D echocardiography can provide additional anatomic information compared to 2D echocardiography. However, because of the relatively poor image quality in current real-time 3D echocardiography,

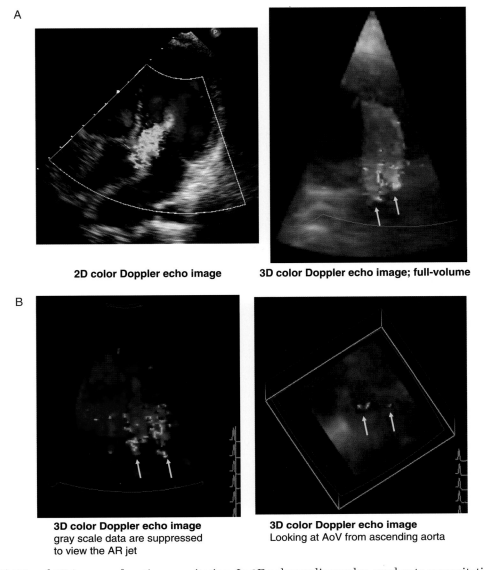

Figure 10.2 (A) 2D and 3D images of aortic regurgitation. In 2D echocardiography, moderate regurgitation is seen with irregular hemispheric acceleration flow. 3D color Doppler echocardiography shows that this patient actually has two regurgitant orifices. (B) Left panel: Gray-scale image is suppressed to view the AR jet. Right panel: The image is rotated as if viewed from within the ascending aorta, two flow jets going through the aortic valve can be observed.

the 3D image alone is not sufficient to make a diagnosis on and observation by 2D echocardiography is a prerequisite. In the full-volume image, the aortic valve is better visualized in the parasternal than in the apical approach. In severe aortic valve calcification, image quality is also low in 2D echocardiography, and visualization of the aortic valve in aortic stenosis is often difficult.

REFERENCES

1. Nemes A, Lagrand WK, McGhie JS et al. Three-dimensional transesophageal echocardiography in the evaluation of aortic valve destruction by endocarditis. J Am Soc Echocardiogr 2006; 19(3): 355.e13–355.e14.

2. Irvine T, Stetten GD, Sachdev V et al. Quantification of aortic regurgitation by real-time 3-dimensional echocardiography in a chronic animal model: computation of aortic regurgitant volume as the difference between left and right ventricular stroke volumes. J Am Soc Echocardiogr 2001; 14(11): 1112–18.

3. Poutanen T, Tikanoja T, Sairanen H, Jokinen E. Normal mitral and aortic valve areas assessed by three- and two-dimensional echocardiography in 168 children and young adults. Pediatr Cardiol 2006; 27(2): 217–25.

4. Miyamoto K, Nakatani S, Kanzaki H et al. Detection of discrete subaortic stenosis by 3-dimensional transesophageal echocardiography. Echocardiography 2005; 22(9): 783–4.

5. Mori Y, Shiota T, Jones M et al. Three-dimensional reconstruction of the color Doppler-imaged vena contracta for quantifying aortic regurgitation: studies in a chronic animal model. Circulation 1999; 99: 1611–17.

6. Fang L, Hsiung MC, Miller AP et al. Assessment of aortic regurgitation by live three-dimensional transthoracic echocardiographic measurements of vena contracta area: usefulness and validation. Echocardiography 2005; 22(9): 775–81.

11 Valvular Heart Disease: Tricuspid Valve

Takeshi Hozumi and Junichi Yoshikawa

TWO-DIMENSIONAL ECHOCARDIOGRAPHY

Images of the tricuspid valve

Because the tricuspid valve is complex both in its anatomy and motion, multiple cross-sectional images should be visualized for comprehensive recognition of the valve. In a parasternal short-axis view at the level of the aortic valve, the septal and anterior leaflets are seen (Figure 11.1). In an apical 4-chamber view, the septal and anterior leaflets of the tricuspid valve are visualized (Figure 11.2). For visualization of the posterior leaflet of the tricuspid valve, the right ventricular inflow tract view should be obtained by medial angulation of the transducer in the parasternal approach (Figure 11.3). In standard two-dimensional (2D) echocardiography, however, it is difficult to visualize all three leaflets in one view. Thus, mental reconstruction of the entire tricuspid valve is necessary from various 2D images.

Tricuspid regurgitation and geometry of the tricuspid valve

Functional tricuspid regurgitation commonly occurs in patients with left-sided valve disease and left ventricular (LV) dysfunction.[1,2] It has been suggested that tricuspid annular dilatation and tethering of the leaflets of the tricuspid valve are important changes in the tricuspid valve geometry in patients with functional tricuspid regurgitation.[3-5] Tricuspid annuloplasty is recommended for the treatment of functional tricuspid regurgitation as a standard surgical procedure at the time of left-sided heart surgery to decrease the postoperative morbidity and mortality because of significant tricuspid regurgitation.[6-8] Although an annuloplasty ring is commonly used in this surgical procedure, residual tricuspid regurgitation commonly occurs. One major reason for this unsatisfactory result may be inadequate knowledge of the three-dimensional (3D) geometry of the tricuspid valve. The rings commonly used for tricuspid annuloplasty were originally formed in a single plane for the mitral valve,[9-11] however the tricuspid annulus may have a non-planar geometry. Although tricuspid diameter, tricuspid tethering distance, and area have been evaluated (Figure 11.4), standard 2D echocardiography produces only a limited recognition of the 3D geometry of the tricuspid valve.

THREE-DIMENSIONAL ECHOCARDIOGRAPHY

Three-dimensional images of the tricuspid valve

Recently developed new real-time 3D echocardiography using a new matrix-array transducer provides more realistic images of tricuspid valve geometry compared with those by conventional 2D echocardiography. In addition, the short-axis view of the

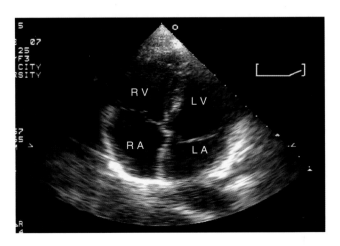

Figure 11.1 Parasternal short-axis view at the level of the aortic valve. LV, left ventricle; RV, right ventricle; LA, left atrium; RA, right atrium.

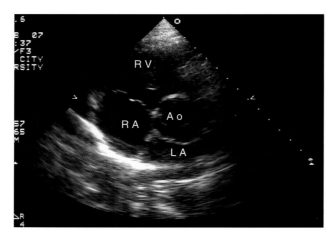

Figure 11.2 Apical 4-chamber view. LA, left atrium; RA, right atrium; RV, right ventricle; Ao, aorta.

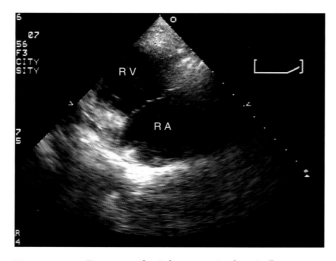

Figure 11.3 Parasternal right ventricular inflow tract view. RA, right atrium; RV, right ventricle.

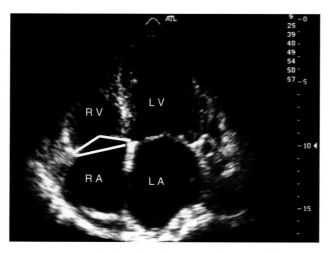

Figure 11.4 Apical 4-chamber view showing the measurement of tricuspid annular diameter, tricuspid tethering distance, and area. LA, left atrium; RA, right atrium; LV, left ventricle; RV, right ventricle.

tricuspid valve, which has not been visualized in 2D echocardiography, can be obtained with good image quality. In real-time 3D echocardiography, images are usually acquired from the apical window in full volume mode for the entire cardiac image data. Two reference 2D images are displayed on the screen, helping the operator to position the region of interest with all targets being covered by the imaging volume. After the reference images have been visualized, such as by apical 4- and 2-chamber views, full-volume datasets of the tricuspid valve are acquired. Four conical subvolumes of approximately 20° × 80° are scanned during 4 to 7 heart beats without the transducer being moved. Under the triggering of the R-wave on the electrocardiogram, the four subvolumes are acquired, automatically integrated, and entire pyramidal datasets of approximately 80° × 80° are obtained. Figure 11.5 shows 3D images of a normal tricuspid valve obtained by real-time 3D echocardiography. All three leaflets of the tricuspid valve are clearly visualized in the 3D images seen from the right ventricle. Figure 11.6 shows the same view of the tricuspid valve in a patient with tricuspid regurgitation. In these 3D images, dilatation of the tricuspid annulus and loss of coaptation of the three tricuspid leaflets are clearly visualized. These images should be helpful for recognition of the pathology of the tricuspid valve in patients with tricuspid regurgitation.

Three-dimensional analysis of tricuspid geometry

Regarding the mitral valve, 3D analysis from multiple cross-sectional images has been applied to the investigation of the non-planar geometry of the valve in earlier reports.[12–15] Although the tricuspid annular size during the cardiac cycle was evaluated using a rotational 2D echocardiographic technique,[3] the non-planar geometry has not been fully investigated. Recently, the 3D geometry of the tricuspid valve has been analyzed with custom-made software[16,17] for the analysis of 3D echocardiographic data obtained from new real-time 3D echocardiography.[18] Figure 11.7 shows real-time 3D images made with the customized software, demonstrating the process of tracing the tricuspid annulus. To acquire the 3D geometry of the tricuspid annulus, the location of eight annulus points should be pinpointed throughout a cardiac cycle from four cross-sectional planes rotated at 45° about a fixed rotational axis. Figure 11.8 shows reconstructed 3D images of the tricuspid annulus in a healthy volunteer and also in a patient with functional tricuspid regurgitation. In this report, the non-planar and non-single-plane structure of the tricuspid annulus was observed both in healthy subjects and in patients with tricuspid regurgitation. In patients with functional tricuspid regurgitation,

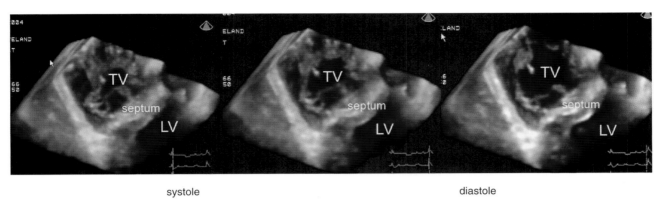

systole   diastole

Figure 11.5   3D images of the tricuspid valve obtained from a healthy subject. LV, left ventricle; TV, tricuspid valve; MV, mitral valve; A, anterior leaflet; P, posterior; S, septum.

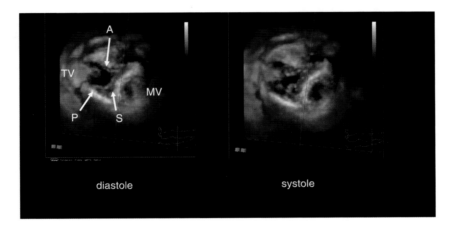

diastole   systole

Figure 11.6   3D images of the tricuspid valve obtained from a patient with severe tricuspid regurgitation. TV, tricuspid valve; MV, mitral valve; A, anterior leaflet; P, posterior; S, septum.

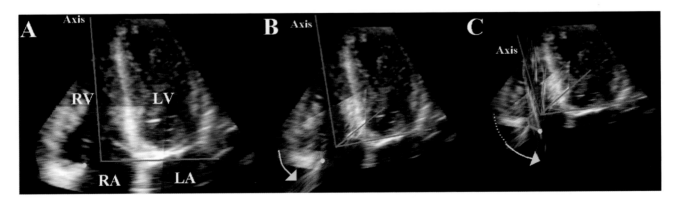

Figure 11.7   Real-time 3D echocardiograms showing the process of tracing the tricuspid annulus. In the cross-sectional plane passing through the middle of the septum, the lateral portion of the tricuspid annulus is manually marked (yellow point) (A). The cross-sectional plane is rotated around the center of the axis (red line) at 45° intervals to mark the posterolateral portion of the tricuspid annulus (yellow point) (B). Then the posterior portion of the tricuspid annulus is marked in the cross-sectional plane rotated 90° from the original position (C). Reproduced from Fukuda et al.[18]

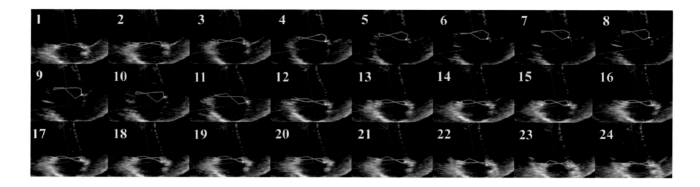

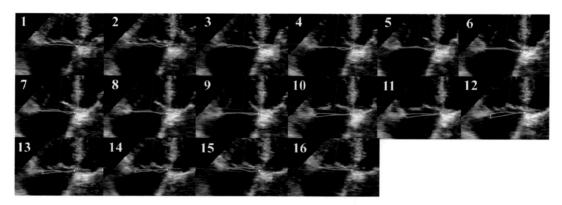

Figure 11.8 3D geometry of the tricuspid annulus in a healthy subject (upper panel) and in a patient with functional tricuspid regurgitation (lower panel) during one cardiac cycle. The dynamic motion of the tricuspid annulus is demonstrated by sequential still images. Composites of still frames start from end-systole in both upper and lower panels. The unique 3D structure of the tricuspid annulus is shown throughout a cardiac cycle in a healthy subject; it was more planar in patients with tricuspid regurgitation. Reproduced from Fukuda et al.[18]

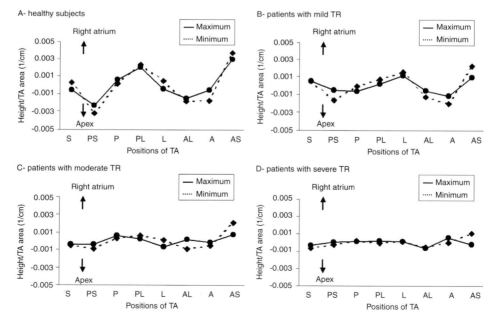

Figure 11.9 Averaged, normalized, localized height of each of the 8 points in healthy subjects (A) and in patients with mild (B), moderate (C), and severe (D) tricuspid regurgitation (TR). A, anterior; AL, anterolateral; AS, anteroseptal; L, lateral; P, posterior; PL, posterolateral; PS, posteroseptal; S, septum; TA, tricuspid annlus. Reproduced from Fukuda et al.[18]

a more circular tricuspid annulus shape was observed because of dilatation of the annulus in the septal to lateral and posteroseptal to anterolateral directions. This study has shown that the more severe the tricuspid regurgitation, the more planar the tricuspid annulus (Figure 11.9). In this analysis, the highest point of the tricuspid annulus was in the anteroseptal segment, and the lowest point toward the right ventricular apex from the right atrium was the posteroseptal segment.

The geometry of the tricuspid annulus appears to be different from the saddle-shaped mitral annulus.[12-15] We may have to consider this point in tricuspid annuloplasty in patients with tricuspid regurgitation. Based on the results of 3D analysis in healthy subjects, an optimal physiologic ring shape could be developed for tricuspid annuloplasty. The use of such a ring may then help to reduce residual tricuspid regurgitation in patients after tricuspid annuloplasty.

REFERENCES

1. Braunwald NS, Ross J Jr, Morrow AG. Conservative management of tricuspid regurgitation in patients undergoing mitral valve replacement. Circulation 1967; 35: I63–9.

2. Nath J, Foster E, Heidenreich PA. Impact of tricuspid regurgitation on long-term survival. J Am Coll Cardiol 2004; 43: 405–9.

3. Tei C, Pilgrim JP, Shah PM, Ormiston JA, Wong M. The tricuspid valve annulus: study of size and motion in normal subjects and in patients with tricuspid regurgitation. Circulation 1982; 66: 665–71.

4. Ubago JL, Figueroa A, Ochoteco A et al. Analysis of the amount of tricuspid valve annular dilatation required to produce functional tricuspid regurgitation. Am J Cardiol 1983; 52: 155–8.

5. Sagie A, Schwammenthal E, Padial LR et al. Determinants of functional tricuspid regurgitation in incomplete tricuspid valve closure: Doppler color flow study of 109 patients. J Am Coll Cardiol 1994; 24: 446–53.

6. Carpentier A, Deloche A, Hanania G et al. Surgical management of acquired tricuspid valve disease. J Thorac Cardiovasc Surg 1974; 67: 53–65.

7. King RM, Schaff HV, Danielson GK et al. Surgery for tricuspid regurgitation late after mitral valve replacement. Circulation 1984; 70(Suppl II): II-193–7.

8. Frater R. Tricuspid insufficiency. J Thorac Cardiovasc Surg 2001; 122: 427–9.

9. Carpentier A, Deloche A, Dauptain J et al. A new reconstructive operation for correction of mitral and tricuspid insufficiency. J Thorac Cardiovasc Surg 1971; 61: 1–13.

10. Unger-Graeber B, Lee RT, Sutton MS et al. Doppler echocardiographic comparison of the Carpentier and Duran annuloplasty rings versus no ring after mitral valve repair for mitral regurgitation. Am J Cardiol 1991; 67: 517–19.

11. McCarthy JF, Cosgrove DM 3rd. Tricuspid valve repair with the Cosgrove–Edwards annuloplasty system. Ann Thorac Surg 1997; 64: 267–8.

12. Ormiston JA, Shah PM, Tei C, Wong M. Size and motion of the mitral valve annulus in man, I: a two-dimensional echocardiographic method and findings in normal subjects. Circulation 1981; 64: 113–20.

13. Levine RA, Handschumacher MD, Sanfilippo AJ et al. Three-dimensional echocardiographic reconstruction of the mitral valve, with implications for the diagnosis of mitral valve prolapse. Circulation 1989; 80: 589–98.

14. Glasson JR, Komeda MK, Daughters GT et al. Three-dimensional regional dynamics of the normal mitral annulus during left ventricular ejection. J Thorac Cardiovasc Surg 1996; 111: 574–85.

15. Kwan J, Qin JX, Popovic ZB et al. Geometric changes of mitral annulus assessed by real-time 3-dimensional echocardiography: becoming enlarged and less nonplanar in the anteroposterior direction during systole in proportion to global left ventricular systolic function. J Am Soc Echocardiogr 2004; 17: 1179–84.

16. Saracino G, Greenberg NL, Shiota T et al. Fast interactive real-time volume rendering of real-time three dimensional echocardiography: an implementation for low-end computers. Comput Cardiol 2002; 29: 613–16.

17. Qin JX, Shiota T, Tsujino H et al. Mitral annular motion as a surrogate for left ventricular ejection fraction: real-time

18. Fukuda S, Saracino G, Matsumura Y et al. Three-dimensional geometry of the tricuspid annulus in healthy subjects and in patients with functional tricuspid regurgitation: a real-time, 3-dimensional echocardiographic study. Circulation 2006; 114(Suppl I): I-492–8.

12 Hypertrophic Cardiomyopathy

Marta Sitges, Carles Paré and Takahiro Shiota

Hypertrophic cardiomyopathy is a cardiovascular disease caused by a genetic disorder in one of at least the 10 genes that encode the proteins of the cardiac sarcomere. This disease has a unique potential for clinical presentation during any phase of life from infancy to old age and may be expressed in a wide range of phenotypic forms, from severe symmetric left ventricular hypertrophy to massive hypertrophy of asymmetric distribution.

Physiopathologic mechanisms underlying hypertrophic cardiomyopathy are complex and not clearly understood, but include dynamic left ventricular outflow obstruction, mitral regurgitation, and diastolic dysfunction. These may all lead to shortness of breath and limited functional capacity, angina, and syncope; however, although most patients are asymptomatic throughout their lives, there is a risk for sudden cardiac death probably associated with arrhythmia and progression to advanced heart failure with left ventricular systolic dysfunction. The main causes of adverse clinical outcome are shown in Table 12.1.

Diagnosis of hypertrophic cardiomyopathy is now mainly based on cardiac imaging methods, including two-dimensional (2D) echocardiography, MRI, and multislice CT scanning. Left ventricular thickening is associated with a non-dilated cavity with hyperdynamic motion and, usually, systolic chamber obliteration. Typically, the diagnosis is made on the presence of a maximal left ventricular wall thickness of at least 15 mm in the absence of any other disease capable of inducing such a degree of left ventricular hypertrophy noted by 2D echocardiography.[1]

Hypertrophic cardiomyopathy can be classified into various hemodynamic subgroups. Patients may present with non-obstructive or obstructive disease; the latter may be even subclassified into latent or provocable (resting gradient < 30 mmHg and > 30 mmHg after provocation) and resting obstructive hypertrophic cardiomyopathy (resting gradient > 30 mmHg).[1]

Two-dimensional echocardiography has been classically the most commonly used imaging technique to evaluate hypertrophic cardiomyopathy. Recent advances in three-dimensional (3D) echocardiography have brought this technique to the clinical field of hypertrophic cardiomyopathy. Because of the abnormal geometry of the hypertrophic ventricle, 3D echo may be a unique, potentially indispensable imaging tool in patients with hypertropic cardiomyopathy.

M-MODE ECHOCARDIOGRAPHY

M-mode echocardiography was the first echocardiographic technique used for the diagnosis of this disease. Typically, an M-mode scan through the left ventricle in the parasternal long axis view allows the detection of a thickened wall (> 15 mm) and a reduced cavity of the left ventricle. The hypertrophy can be of concentric or asymmetric distribution, usually affecting the septal wall (Figures 12.1 and 12.2), with a septal to posterior wall ratio > 1.5:1. Care must be taken when using M-mode to avoid

Table 12.1 Causes of adverse outcome in hypertrophic cardiomyopathy
Sudden death/ventricular arrhythmia
Refractory heart failure symptoms
LVOT obstruction
Diastolic dysfunction
Systolic dysfunction (left ventricular remodeling)
Complications related to atrial fibrillation (embolic stroke)
LVOT: left ventricular outflow tract.

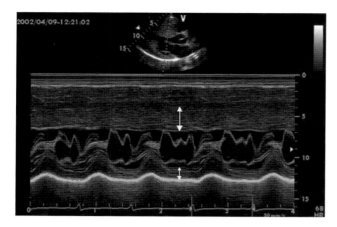

Figure 12.1 M-mode scan across the basal level of the left ventricle in the parasternal long-axis view showing asymmetric septal hypertrophy with severe hypertrophy of the septum (large arrow) and mild hypertrophy of the posterior wall (small arrow).

oblique cuts of the interventricular septum or incorrect identification of echoes from the right side of the septum that may lead to overestimation of left ventricular hypertrophy. M-mode echocardiography can also determine the existence, degree, and duration of an abnormal anterior movement of the mitral valve during systole (SAM), related to several factors such as abnormalities in the mitral valve apparatus (i.e. posterior to anterior leaflet mismatch and abnormal disposition of the subvalvular apparatus), reduced left ventricular outflow tract dimensions, and the Venturi effect of the abnormally accelerated left ventricular outflow. The duration of the contact of the mitral valve with the septal wall allows the classification of the severity of the SAM,[2] given the high temporal resolution of

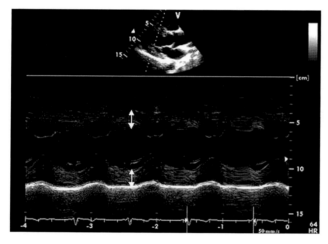

Figure 12.2 M-mode scan across the basal level of the left ventricle in the parasternal long-axis view showing symmetric hypertrophy with severe hypertrophy of both the septum and the posterior wall (arrows) with a ratio close to 1:1.

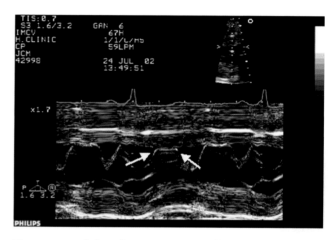

Figure 12.4 M-mode scan across the mitral valve in the parasternal long-axis view demonstrating anterior displacement of the mitral valve (SAM) during the whole systole with complete contact of the valve and the septum (arrows).

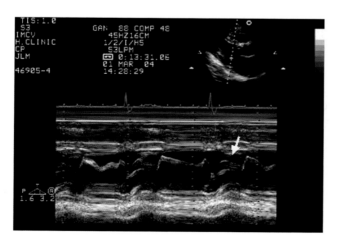

Figure 12.3 M-mode scan across the mitral valve in the parasternal long-axis view demonstrating anterior displacement of the mitral valve during systole (SAM), but without complete septal contact (arrow).

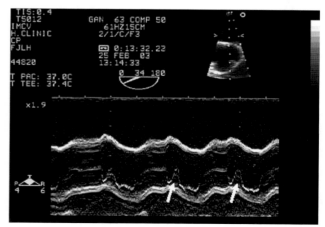

Figure 12.5 M-mode scan across the aortic valve guided by 2D transesophageal echocardiography in a patient with hypertrophic obstructive cardiomyopathy depicting abnormal early closure of the aortic valve during mid-systole (arrows).

M-mode scans across the mitral valve in the parasternal long axis (Figures 12.3 and 12.4). Additionally, M-mode interrogation of the aortic valve leaflets provides indirect hemodynamic information about the existence of left ventricular outflow obstruction as the early closing of an otherwise normally appearing aortic valve can be detected during midsystole (Figure 12.5). This mid-systolic closure or notching of the aortic valve must be differentiated from other causes of severe left ventricular hypertrophy such as the presence of a subaortic fixed stenosis (subaortic membrane), where the abnormal closure of the aortic valve occurs in early systole, or a valvular aortic stenosis, where the valve does not open properly throughout the whole systole and thickening of the aortic leaflets is present.

TWO-DIMENSIONAL ECHOCARDIOGRAPHY

Two-dimensional echocardiography provides a powerful tool to evaluate patients with hypertrophic cardiomyopathy with more anatomic information of the whole cardiac cavities (Figure 12.6). Two-dimensional echocardiography allows a better understanding of the distribution of the hypertrophy

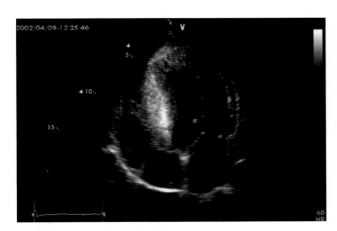

Figure 12.6 Two-dimensional apical 4-chamber view depicting severe left ventricular hypertrophy involving the whole septal wall and the apex. The lateral wall and right ventricle are much less affected.

Table 12.2 Distribution of hypertrophic cardiomyopathy in the left ventricle

Asymmetric:	
Septal	90%
Mid-ventricular	1%
Apical	3%
Posterolateral wall	1%
Symmetric (concentric)	5%

than M-mode echo, especially in those rare presentations affecting other localizations than the septal or the posterior wall such as the left ventricular inferior or lateral wall[3] (Table 12.2). The distribution

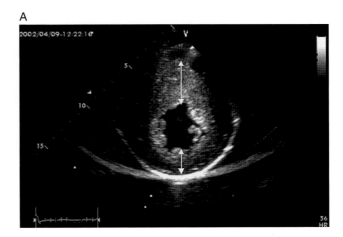

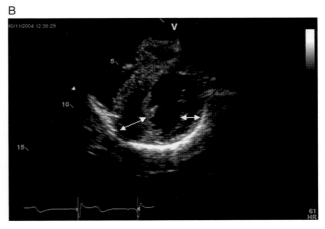

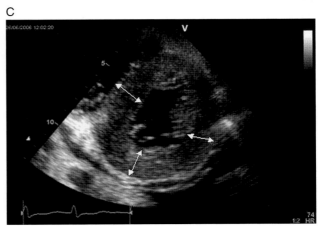

Figure 12.7 2D short-axis view of the left ventricle at the papillary muscle level demonstrating atypical asymmetric left ventricular hypertrophy affecting predominantly the anterior septum (A, large arrow) or more infrequently the posterior septum and the inferior wall (B, large arrow). (C) 2D short-axis view of the left ventricle at the papillary muscle level demonstrating typical concentric left ventricular hypertrophy with similar wall thickness at the septum, posterior and lateral wall (arrows).

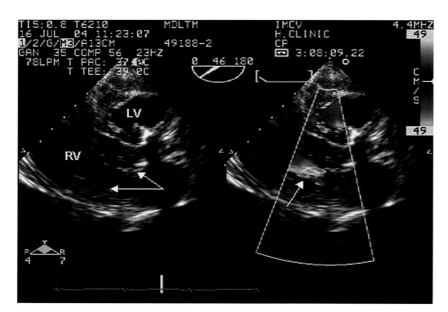

Figure 12.8 Two-dimensional transesophageal echocardiography: short-axis view of the left (LV) and right ventricle (RV) depicting right ventricular hypertrophy (arrows) that induces outflow obstruction as suggested by the systolic color flow turbulence seen in the right panel (arrow).

of left ventricular hypertrophy may be well determined by the use of 2D echo in the short-axis view of the left ventricle, where the whole transversal section of the left ventricular wall and cavity can be examined in most cases (Figure 12.7). From this view, this technique may also be able to detect right ventricular involvement (Figure 12.8). Finally, 2D echocardiography may be of particular utility to diagnose infrequent forms of apical distribution, especially with the use of contrast agents. This phenotypic expression of the disease is less frequent but has a high prevalence in Japan. Typically, it is not associated with left ventricular outflow tract obstruction but with cavity obliteration showing a 'spade-like' left ventricular appearance in systole[4] (Figure 12.9). For this reason, it has to be differentiated from other diseases that may occupy the apex such as the hypereosinophilic syndrome or the presence of an intraventricular thrombus. Other rare presentations of hypertrophic cardiomyopathy include those affecting the posterolateral left ventricular wall and those of mid-ventricular location with cavity obstruction at this level.[5]

In cases of symmetric, concentric left ventricular hypertrophy, hypertrophic cardiomyopathy has to be differentiated from that 'physiologic' left ventricular hypertrophy related to physical training (athlete's heart); in the case of severe concentric hypertrophy, a differential diagnosis has to be made with infiltrative disease such as amyloidotic cardiomyopathy.

In an upper level at the short-axis view, the left ventricular outflow may be sometimes evaluated with virtual occlusion during systole in those cases of concomitant left ventricular outflow obstruction.

Also, from the apical views, 2D echocardiography facilitates evaluation of the distribution of the

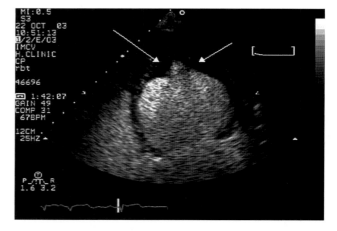

Figure 12.9 Contrast-enhanced 2D echocardiography: 4-chamber apical view of the left ventricle which shows a typical 'spade-like' appearance due to the presence of apical hypertrophy. The thickness of the basal and mid-segments of the left ventricle is normal while the apex has collapsed due to the wall hypertrophy existing at this level (arrows).

left ventricular hypertrophy that may affect mostly the basal septum but can also involve the whole septal wall. In elderly patients, left ventricular hypertrophy is usually located at the level of the basal septum, which maintains its normal curvature leading to an ovoid-shaped left ventricular cavity (Figure 12.10). On the other hand, in younger patients, hypertrophy usually involves the whole septal wall, which shows a convex curvature toward the cavity (reversed abnormal septal curvature), leading to a crescent-shaped left ventricular cavity (Figure 12.6).

In those patients with obstructive disease (around 25% of patients with hypertrophic cardiomyopathy), left ventricular hypertrophy is

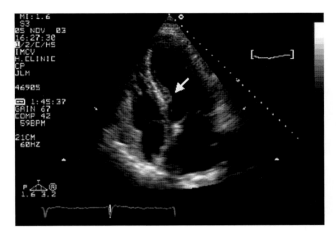

Figure 12.10 2D echo 4-chamber apical view of a 70-year-old patient with hypertrophic cardiomyopathy affecting mainly the basal septum (arrow), where the thickness was 17 mm, while in the other left ventricular segments it was 13 mm (anterior wall) and 12 mm (posterolateral wall).

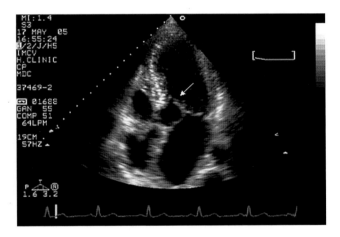

Figure 12.11 2D 4-chamber apical view showing systolic contact of the mitral valve with the septum due to the anterior movement of the former during systole.

often accompanied by SAM noticeable with 2D scans by the systolic contact of the mitral valve and the septal wall (Figure 12.11). SAM may be caused by the anterior movement of the anterior leaflet (10%) or the posterior leaflet (31%) or, more commonly, both (58%). In a few cases, systolic anterior movement is only noted at the chordal structure, which usually does not translate into significant obstruction. The mitral leaflets are significantly longer and mismatch between the anterior and posterior leaflet has also been demonstrated in patients with obstructive hypertrophic cardiomyopathy.[6] Lesions in the mitral valve are also frequently associated with hypertrophic cardiomyopathy (around 20%) and can be evaluated with 2D echocardiography; accordingly, calcification of the mitral

annulus, thickening of the valves, and, less frequently, leaflet prolapse can be detected.[7]

Left atrial dimension, an index of chronic diastolic dysfunction, and mitral regurgitation, which are both usually observed in these patients, can also be assessed with 2D echocardiography, mainly from the apical views. Finally, 2D echocardiography permits the estimation of left ventricular systolic function as in any cardiac disease. In most cases, the hypertrophied left ventricle moves hyperdynamically in systole resulting in cavity obliteration, clearly seen from all parasternal and apical views. However, few patients develop severe systolic dysfunction[8,9] which can be detected by 2D echocardiography during follow-up, even requiring heart transplantation in rare situations.

COLOR DOPPLER ECHOCARDIOGRAPHY

Color Doppler 2D echocardiography detects the presence of a turbulent flow in the left ventricular outflow tract in the case of left intraventricular obstruction (Figure 12.12). Obstruction in hypertrophic cardiomyopathy may occur at three levels: left ventricular outflow tract, mid-ventricular, and apical, being the most frequent obstruction at the outflow tract (Table 12.3). However, distinguishing the three levels of obstruction may be sometimes challenging. The presence of a flow convergence area in the left ventricular outflow tract points to the existence of obstruction at this level, probably due to an associated SAM, while visualization of a turbulent flow in the mid or apical cavity may help in the diagnosis of these less frequent forms of hypertrophic cardiomyopathy.[10] Mid-ventricular obstruction may also develop secondary to apical myocardial infarction in the presence of angiographically normal coronary arteries or in patients with coronary artery disease and diffuse involvement of ventricular hypertrophy.[9,11]

In addition, color Doppler diagnoses the presence of mitral regurgitation as a consequence of the SAM and/or the coexistence of organic valve disease.[12,13] The quantification of mitral regurgitation in the presence of left ventricular outflow tract obstruction may be cumbersome and of especial difficulty as both turbulent flows merge together, making it difficult to clearly visualize the flow convergence of the mitral regurgitant jet. Additionally, the mitral regurgitant jet is usually eccentric and directed postero-laterally to the left atrium (Figure 12.12).

PULSED AND CONTINUOUS WAVE DOPPLER

Pulsed wave Doppler cannot always be reliably applied in patients with hypertrophic cardiomyopathy as flow velocity is increased in the left

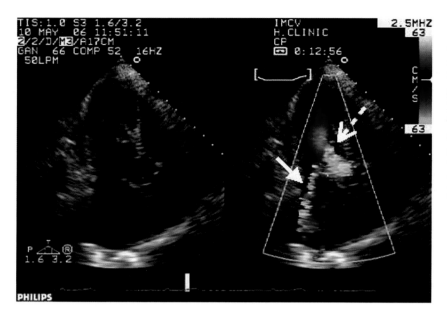

Figure 12.12   2D long-axis apical view of a patient with obstructive hypertrophic cardiomyopathy. Right and left panel show the same 3-chamber apical view, respectively, without and with color Doppler, respectively. In the left panel, color Doppler shows turbulent flow both at the left ventricular outflow tract (broken arrow), suggesting the presence of a significant increase in flow velocity at this level, and mitral regurgitation with an eccentric jet directed posterolaterally (closed arrow).

Table 12.3   Causes of left ventricular systolic obstruction
Obstruction at the left ventricular outflow tract:
Septal hypertrophy and SAM
Discrete subaortic stenosis
Mitral valve replacement (position of the strut)
Mitral valve repair with SAM
Anomalous mitral valve apparatus:
○ abnormal papillary muscles
○ mitral accessory tissue
Mid-ventricular obstruction:
Mid-ventricular hypertrophic cardiomyopathy
Apical hypertrophic cardiomyopathy
Apical myocardial infarction with hyperdynamic contraction of the basal and mid-ventricular segments
Cavity obliteration:
Apical hypertrophic cardiomyopathy (apical cavity obliteration)
Hyperdynamic state
Hypovolemia
Concentric left ventricular hypertrophy (secondary to hypertension, aortic stenosis)

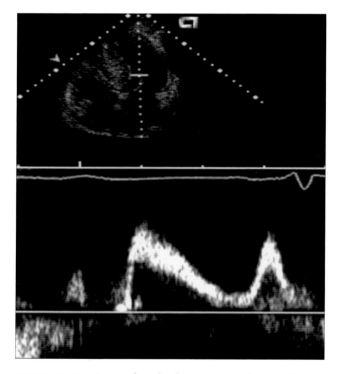

Figure 12.13   Spectral pulsed-wave Doppler of the left ventricular inflow in a patient with hypertrophic cardiomyopathy, showing early (E wave) to late (A wave) peak diastolic velocities with a ratio (E/A) of approximately 1, but with a prolonged deceleration time of the E wave (290 ms), suggesting an abnormal relaxation with a pseudonormal diastolic pattern due to increased filling pressures.

ventricle cavity and aliasing occurs. However, in the presence of left ventricular or mid-cavity obstruction, pulsed wave Doppler may be of particular interest, allowing the detection of the level at which the obstruction is produced by mapping flow velocity from the apex to the outflow tract.[14] Additionally, pulsed wave Doppler is useful to evaluate diastolic left ventricular function, mostly impaired in patients with hypertrophic cardiomyopathy.[15] Abnormal,

delayed relaxation is the most frequent diastolic pattern found. Pseudonormalization is also often seen in patients with left ventricular outflow tract obstruction and secondary mitral regurgitation with increased atrial pressure (Figure 12.13). Also, a restrictive pattern may be seen as an effect of

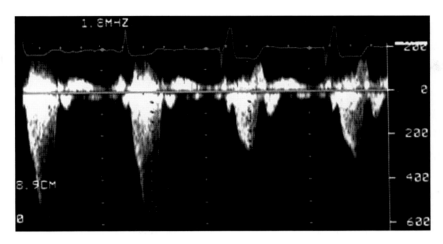

Figure 12.14 Continuous wave spectral Doppler scan demonstrating the presence of two high-velocity flows in systole, the highest and more round-shaped corresponding to mitral regurgitation (left side in the figure) and the other, typically dagger-shaped corresponding to the obstructive gradient in the left ventricular outflow tract (right side in the figure).

increased chamber stiffness causing both rapid atrial–ventricular pressure equilibration (rapid deceleration time) and compensatory increases in left atrial pressure (increased E wave velocity).[16–19] Finally, pulsed wave Doppler of the left ventricular inflow combined with velocities of the mitral annulus determined with pulsed tissue Doppler may also provide accurate estimates of left ventricular filling pressures.[20,21]

Continuous wave Doppler is an essential tool for the complete evaluation of patients with hypertrophic cardiomyopathy. It allows the estimation of the severity of intraventricular obstruction. Excellent correlation has been demonstrated between pressure gradients determined from continuous wave Doppler and cardiac catheterization in different subsets of patients with hypertrophic cardiomyopathy.[10,22–24] Typically, the spectral continuous wave Doppler shows a dagger-shaped gradient across the left ventricular outflow tract (Figure 12.14) that may be confounded with the spectral signal of mitral regurgitation, usually more round-shaped, but sometimes really difficult to differentiate from. Usually, mitral regurgitant flow reaches peak velocities of about 5 or 6 m/s, while intraventricular obstruction rarely overcomes those values.[25] It is important to interrogate the left ventricular outflow tract with continuous wave Doppler in both the resting state and after a provocation maneuver, either Valsalva or handgrip maneuver, physical exercise, pharmacologic stress, or amyl nitrite administration. Evaluation of the intraventricular gradient with this technique is the main imaging tool to evaluate the efficacy of a given therapy in patients with hypertrophic cardiomyopathy. However, its unpredictable variability even throughout the same day is also reported.[26]

As previously mentioned, intraventricular obstruction in hypertrophic cardiomyopathy may take place at three levels and their differentiation may be not easy. With continuous wave Doppler, each has the typical concave 'dagger-shaped' systolic Doppler wave form, but the highest velocities

Table 12.4   Three-dimensional echocardiography in hypertrophic cardiomyopathy
Distribution of LV hypertrophy
LV mass assessment
Assessment of left atrium
Evaluation of LVOT
Effect of interventional therapies
LV: left ventricular; LVOT: left ventricular outflow tract.

generally occur with left outflow tract obstruction and the peak velocity occurs later in systole for mid-ventricular and in cavity obliteration.[10,23]

ROLE OF THREE-DIMENSIONAL ECHOCARDIOGRAPHY IN HYPERTROPHIC CARDIOMYOPATHY

Distribution and quantification of left ventricular hypertrophy

Table 12.4 summarizes the potential utility of three-dimensional echocardiography in patients with hypertrophic cardiomyopathy. Three-dimensional echocardiography provides an absolute volume of the left and right ventricles and the distribution of hypertrophy, particularly in those asymmetric presentations or in the apical form[27] (Figure 12.15).

Post-processing of the 3D images allows acquisition of any given slice across the left ventricle cavity without the problem of misalignment typically observed with M-mode and 2D echocardiography that may show tangential slices of the left ventricular wall giving, therefore, the false diagnosis of wall hypertrophy. Also in this regard, 3D techniques may allow the location and quantification of the maximum thickness of the myocardium. This parameter has been shown to have prognostic

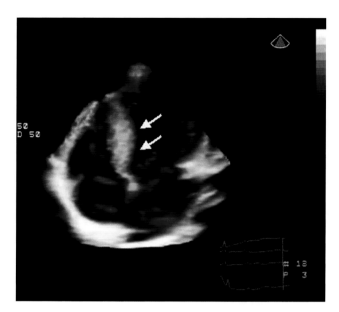

Figure 12.15 Transthoracic three-dimensional echocardiography from the apical view showing asymmetric septal hypertrophy (arrows).

implications in terms of risk of cardiac sudden death.[1]

Left and right ventricular volumes can be accurately estimated with 3D echo according to several studies that have compared the results of 3D echo and magnetic resonance imaging, phantoms, or electromagnetically derived volumes.[28–30] The abnormal geometry of the cavity of a hypertrophied ventricle may be a good substrate for evaluation with 3D echocardiography as geometric assumptions are not needed and, consequently, eliminated (Figure 12.16).

Similarly, ventricular mass may also be measured with more reliability and accuracy by the use of this technique.[31]

Different studies have validated the estimation of left ventricular mass with M-mode or 2D echocardiography on post-mortem specimens, based on different geometric models. However, these geometric assumptions may not always hold true in the case of hypertrophic cardiomyopathy, often leading to errors in the calculation of left ventricular mass. Early reconstructive 3D echocardiographic techniques demonstrated that accuracy was improved and reproducibility increased for left ventricular mass measurement with the use of 3D echo in comparison with M-mode and 2D echo.[32,33] More recently, real-time 3D echocardiography has also shown the ability to increase the accuracy of left ventricular mass estimation in vivo and in vitro with a SEE of 8.5 g.[31,34] Accuracy was especially improved in those cases of asymmetric left ventricles. With developing technologies to improve spatial resolution and

visualization, real-time 3D echocardiography may become the imaging technique of choice for left ventricular mass determination in clinical studies looking at hypertrophy regression in hypertrophic cardiomyopathy, arterial hypertension, or aortic stenosis.

Evaluation of left atrial size

Assessment of left atrial size and function may be of importance in patients with hypertrophic cardiomyopathy for several reasons. As previously mentioned, it may be an index of the severity and chronicity of both mitral regurgitation and diastolic dysfunction.[35,36] Also, it may constitute a risk factor for atrial fibrillation that usually induces hemodynamic and clinical worsening of patients with hypertrophic cardiomyopathy. Similar to what has been formerly discussed for the evaluation of the left ventricular volumes and mass, the 3D methodology avoids any geometric assumption, making it a method of choice to measure left atrial volume[37] (Figure 12.17). By the use of real-time 3D echocardiography it has been proved that left ventricular thickness is the most important determinant of left atrial dilation, followed by left ventricular end-diastolic pressure and outflow tract obstruction.[38]

Left atrial size has been demonstrated to decrease after septal reduction therapies, either surgical myectomy or the more recently introduced percutaneous transcoronary septal myocardial ablation (PTSMA).[17,36] Three-dimensional echocardiography may also become a useful tool for the evaluation of the results of these techniques and their impact on left atrial size and function.

Evaluation of left ventricular outflow tract area

As previously mentioned, some patients with hypertrophic cardiomyopathy have obstruction in the left ventricular outflow tract due to narrowing caused by the hypertrophied left ventricle and due to the systolic anterior movement of the mitral valve.[39] Severe left ventricular outflow tract obstruction may contribute to the development of dyspnea, syncope, and angina in these patients.[40] Consequently, treatment of such patients with obstructive hypertrophic cardiomyopathy should be directed to reduce left ventricular outflow obstruction (Figure 12.18). For this purpose, negative inotropic drugs such as beta-blockers or calcium channel blockers have been proposed, with efficacy rates around 70% when maximum titration can be tolerated.[1] Dual-chamber pacing has also been used as an alternative to reduce outflow tract obstruction, with controversial results.[41–43]

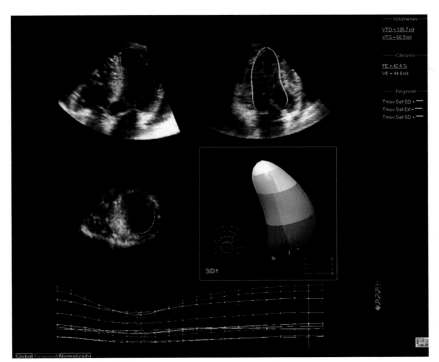

Figure 12.16 Measurement of the left ventricular volume with a dedicated software from transthoracic 3D echocardiography scans. Segmental volumes of the left ventricle throughout the cardiac cycle are shown at the bottom of the figure, while the whole reconstructed left ventricular cavity is shown at the top.

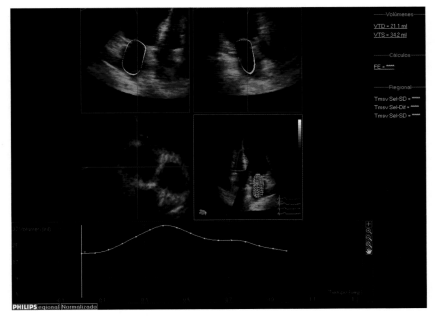

Figure 12.17 Measurement of the left atrial volume with a dedicated software from transthoracic 3D echocardiography scans. The volume of the left atrium throughout the cardiac cycle is shown on the bottom panel, while the whole reconstructed left atrial cavity is shown in a mesh form.

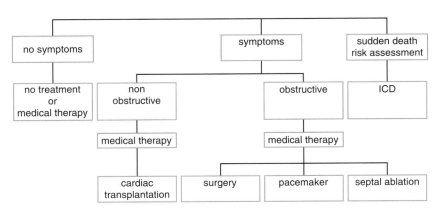

Figure 12.18 Therapeutic algorithm in hypertrophic cardiomyopathy. ICD, implantable cardiac defibrilator.

Both surgical myectomy and PTSMA effectively reduce left ventricular outflow tract obstruction in patients with hypertrophic obstructive cardiomyopathy.[44–48] The former surgically eliminates (direct scission) a piece of the hypertrophied septal muscle while the latter chemically induces necrosis of the basal septal myocardium by the injection of ethanol into one septal coronary artery branch. Significant and sustained reductions in left ventricular outflow tract pressure gradients have been reported after PTSMA, with a reasonable safety profile in long-term follow-up.[48] On the other hand, outcomes are also very good after surgical myectomy in specialized centers, with high rates of abolition of outflow obstruction.[46,49,50]

Measurement of the efficacy of these treatments is usually based on indirect signs of obstruction such as the presence of significant pressure gradients through the left ventricular outflow tract (Figure 12.19). Evaluation of the left ventricular outflow tract anatomy is difficult with 2D image methods due to the complex and 3D nature of the outflow tract anatomy. Three-dimensional imaging techniques such as 3D echocardiography or magnetic resonance imaging theoretically provide better information about this structure and the complex relationship between the mitral valve, the septum, and the left ventricular outflow tract (Figure 12.20). The degree of the outflow obstruction is usually determined by continuous wave Doppler through the left ventricular outflow tract guided by 2D imaging. However, as noted above, concomitant mitral regurgitation may cause uncertainty of this measurement despite typical dagger-shaped

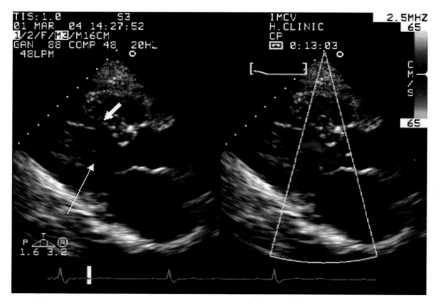

Figure 12.19 Two-dimensional echocardiography in a patient with obstructive hypertrophic cardiomyopathy who underwent percutaneous septal alcohol ablation 6 months previously. Left panel: parasternal long-axis view showing mild anterior displacement of the mitral chordae towards the septum without contacting it (thin arrow) and a focal thinning of the basal septum where the necrosis was chemically induced (thick arrow). Interrogation with color Doppler (right panel) confirms the absence of turbulent flow in the outflow tract and, therefore, the elimination of obstruction at this level.

A
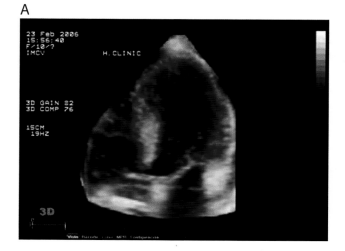

B
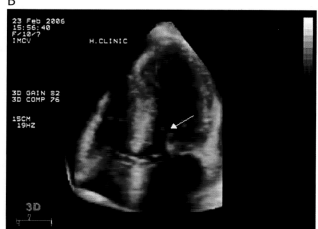

Figure 12.20 Apical view in transthoracic 3D echocardiography exam in end-diastole (A) and mid-systole (B) showing the anterior movement of the mitral valve towards the septum and partially obstructing the left ventricular outflow tract during systole (arrow).

continuous wave Doppler profiles of the left ventricular outflow tract obstruction. In such a patient, direct 3D visualization of the narrowed left ventricular outflow tract area and direct measurement of the area would be of great value to confirm the severity of the outflow obstruction. In addition, when PTSMA or myectomy is performed, direct 3D visualization of the opened or widened left ventricular outflow tract would be not only visually impressive, but also important for knowing the location and extent of the septal reduction.

A few studies have reported the capability of 3D echo to assess the left ventricular outflow tract area.[51,52] It has been proved with reconstructed images from 3D transthoracic echo that patients with hypertrophic cardiomyopathy have a more elliptical left ventricular outflow tract than normal subjects; also, asymmetry of the outflow tract is highest in patients with outflow obstruction at rest, indicating that for a similar cross-sectional area, the asymmetry of the left ventricular outflow tract may play a role in the presence of significant obstruction.[51,52] Three-dimensional echocardiography can provide precise quantitative assessment of the minimal cross-sectional area of the left ventricular outflow tract as well as of its temporal changes,[53] which is a determinant of systolic outflow obstruction.[54] Accordingly, real-time 3D echocardiographic studies have demonstrated a significant relationship between left ventricular outflow tract areas and pressure gradients.[53,55]

Additionally, with the 3D technique, the location of systolic anterior motion of the mitral valve, which is not constantly produced from the center of the anterior leaflet, can be precisely determined by moving the 2D short-axis plane across the left ventricular outflow tract in the 3D space.[53,55] Two-dimensional echo may underestimate the severity of systolic anterior motion of the mitral valve because of errors in the image plane and misalignment. Recognition of the asymmetry of mitral systolic anterior motion and septal hypertrophy may be of special interest for surgeons in determining the exact location of resection and whether concomitant mitral valve surgery is necessary to eliminate obstruction.

Also, multiplane transesophageal echo with 3D reconstruction provided evidence of a significant increase in the left ventricular outflow tract area in 11 patients undergoing myectomy.[52] With real-time 3D echocardiography these results have been confirmed and, also, an increased outflow tract area has been demonstrated after alcohol septal ablation. Indeed, it was found that although both techniques are effective in reducing left ventricular outflow tract obstruction, the increase in left ventricular outflow tract area was greater for myectomy than alcohol septal ablation.[55] These results are in accordance with other findings showing that the

effect of myectomy on left ventricular outflow tract obstruction may be more definitive than alcohol septal ablation.[47] Therefore, 3D echocardiography should be an imaging technique of choice in patients with obstructive hypertrophic cardiomyopathy to diagnose obstruction and to evaluate the effect of therapies, particularly those involving septal reduction either chemically (alcohol ablation) or mechanically (myectomy). This may even be applied in the operating room, with the epicardial

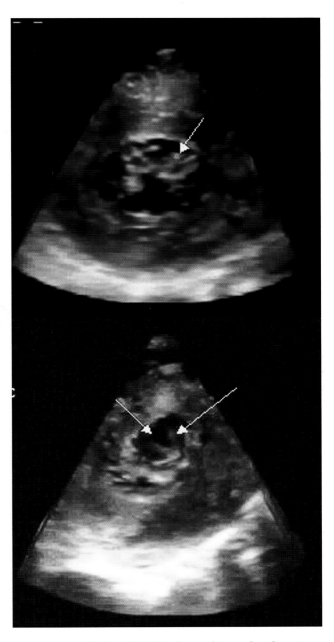

Figure 12.21 Epicardial 3D echocardiography showing a short-axis view of the mitral valve and the left ventricular outflow tract of a patient with obstructive hypertrophic cardiomyopathy undergoing surgical myectomy. Top: before myectomy, the left ventricular outflow tract is narrowed (arrow). Bottom: after surgery, the left ventricular outflow tract has significantly increased (arrows).

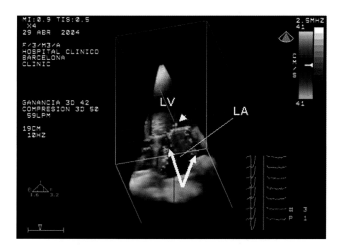

Figure 12.22 Transthoracic 3D color Doppler echocardiography showing an eccentric regurgitant flow: there is a double jet mitral regurgitation (arrows) with a unique flow convergence area (triangle). A plane was found by 3D echo in which all components could be appreciated. LA, left atrium; LV, left ventricle.

approach or with a 3D echo transesophageal probe[56,57] (Figure 12.21). Additionally, early detection of iatrogenic ventricular septal defect could be facilitated intraoperatively with the use of color Doppler 3D echo as an eccentric and tortuous path of the abnormal shunting flow may be detected more easily with this technique.

Assessment of mitral regurgitation

Mitral regurgitation due to systolic anterior movement of the mitral valve generates eccentric regurgitant jets and, as previously mentioned, it is usually difficult to quantify the severity of the regurgitation. Three-dimensional color Doppler echocardiography may be useful to better quantify mitral regurgitant jets in these patients, either by assessment of the full volume of the regurgitant flow or by more accurate visualization and measurement of the flow convergence area.[58–60] Accordingly, real-time 3D color Doppler echo has been shown to provide unique information about the flow convergence zone geometry, resulting in accurate estimates of mitral regurgitant volume and orifice area in experimental models and clinical settings. Three-dimensional color Doppler echo also provides unique information about the origin, direction, and flow pattern of the regurgitant jet (Figure 12.22) and, indeed, several studies have shown a good correlation with angiographic grading of mitral regurgitation.[59–61]

SUMMARY

Echocardiography has played a pivotal role in the diagnosis of hypertrophic cardiomyopathy and in the evaluation of the effect of therapy in patients with obstructive disease. Considering unique abnormalities in cardiac geometry in hypertrophic cardiomyopathy, 3D echocardiography will become a powerful additional tool in evaluating and managing these patients.

ACKNOWLEDGMENTS

We are indebted to Manel Azqueta MD and Victoria Delgado MD for their valuable help in the elaboration of the illustrations.

REFERENCES

1. Maron BJ, McKenna WJ, Danielson GK et al. American College of Cardiology/European Society of Cardiology clinical expert consensus document on hypertrophic cardiomyopathy. A report of the American College of Cardiology Foundation Task Force on Clinical Expert Consensus Documents and the European Society of Cardiology Committee for Practice Guidelines. J Am Coll Cardiol 2003; 42: 1687–713.

2. Gilbert BW, Pollick C, Adelman AG, Wigle ED. Hypertrophic cardiomyopathy: subclassification by M mode echocardiography. Am J Cardiol 1980; 45: 861–72.

3. Maron BJ, Gottdiener JS, Epstein SE. Patterns and significance of distribution of left ventricular hypertrophy in hypertrophic cardiomyopathy. A wide angle, two dimensional echocardiographic study of 125 patients. Am J Cardiol 1981; 48: 418–28.

4. Yamaguchi H, Ishimura T, Nishiyama S et al. Hypertrophic nonobstructive cardiomyopathy with giant negative T waves (apical hypertrophy): ventriculographic and echocardiographic features in 30 patients. Am J Cardiol 1979; 44: 401–12.

5. Falicov RE, Resnekov L, Bharati S, Lev M. Mid-ventricular obstruction: a variant of obstructive cardiomyopathy. Am J Cardiol 1976; 37: 432–7.

6. Schwammenthal E, Nakatani S, He S et al. Mechanism of mitral regurgitation in hypertrophic cardiomyopathy: mismatch of posterior to anterior leaflet length and mobility. Circulation 1998; 98: 856–65.

7. Grigg LE, Wigle ED, Williams WG, Daniel LB, Rakowski H. Transesophageal Doppler echocardiography in obstructive hypertrophic cardiomyopathy: clarification of pathophysiology and importance in intraoperative decision making. J Am Coll Cardiol 1992; 20: 42–52.

8. Spirito P, Maron BJ. Absence of progression of left ventricular hypertrophy in adult patients with hypertrophic cardiomyopathy. J Am Coll Cardiol 1987; 9: 1013–17.

9. Fighali S, Krajcer Z, Edelman S, Leachman RD. Progression of hypertrophic cardiomyopathy into a hypokinetic left ventricle: higher incidence in patients with midventricular obstruction. J Am Coll Cardiol 1987; 9: 288–94.

10. Schwammenthal E, Block M, Schwartzkopff B et al. Prediction of the site and severity of obstruction in hypertrophic cardiomyopathy by color flow mapping and continuous wave Doppler echocardiography. J Am Coll Cardiol 1992; 20: 964–72.

11. Webb JG, Sasson Z, Rakowski H, Liu P, Wigle ED. Apical hypertrophic cardiomyopathy: clinical follow-up and diagnostic correlates. J Am Coll Cardiol 1990; 15: 83–90.

12. Roberts CS, Gertz SD, Klues HG et al. Appearance of or persistence of severe mitral regurgitation without left ventricular outflow obstruction after partial ventricular septal myotomy-myectomy in hypertrophic cardiomyopathy. Am J Cardiol 1991; 68: 1726–8.

13. Rakowski H, Sasson Z, Wigle ED. Echocardiographic and Doppler assessment of hypertrophic cardiomyopathy. J Am Soc Echocardiogr 1988; 1: 31–47.

14. Sasson Z, Yock PG, Hatle LK, Alderman EL, Popp RL. Doppler echocardiographic determination of the pressure gradient in hypertrophic cardiomyopathy. J Am Coll Cardiol 1988; 11: 752–6.

15. Spirito P, Maron BJ, Chiarella F et al. Diastolic abnormalities in patients with hypertrophic cardiomyopathy: relation to magnitude of left ventricular hypertrophy. Circulation 1985; 72: 310–16.

16. Spirito P, Maron BJ. Relation between extent of left ventricular hypertrophy and diastolic filling abnormalities in hypertrophic cardiomyopathy. J Am Coll Cardiol 1990; 15: 808–13.

17. Sitges M, Shiota T, Lever HM et al. Comparison of left ventricular diastolic function in obstructive hypertrophic cardiomyopathy in patients undergoing percutaneous septal alcohol ablation versus surgical myotomy/myectomy. Am J Cardiol 2003; 91: 817–21.

18. Nihoyannopoulos P, Karatasakis G, Frenneaux M, McKenna WJ, Oakley CM. Diastolic function in hypertrophic cardiomyopathy: relation to exercise capacity. J Am Coll Cardiol 1992; 19: 536–40.

19. Elliott PM, Brecker SJ, McKenna WJ. Diastolic dysfunction in hypertrophic cardiomyopathy. Eur Heart J 1998; 19: 1125–7.

20. Nagueh SF, Lakkis NM, Middleton KJ et al. Doppler estimation of left ventricular filling pressures in patients with hypertrophic cardiomyopathy. Circulation 1999; 99: 254–61.

21. Nishimura RA, Appleton CP, Redfield MM et al. Noninvasive Doppler echocardiographic evaluation of left ventricular filling pressures in patients with cardiomyopathies: a simultaneous Doppler echocardiographic and cardiac catheterization study. J Am Coll Cardiol 1996; 28: 1226–33.

22. Stewart WJ, Schiavone WA, Salcedo EE et al. Intraoperative Doppler echocardiography in hypertrophic cardiomyopathy: correlations with the obstructive gradient. J Am Coll Cardiol 1987; 10: 327–35.

23. Panza JA, Petrone RK, Fananapazir L, Maron BJ. Utility of continuous wave Doppler echocardiography in the noninvasive assessment of left ventricular outflow tract pressure gradient in patients with hypertrophic cardiomyopathy. J Am Coll Cardiol 1992; 19: 91–9.

24. Schwammenthal E, Schwartzkopff B, Block M et al. Doppler echocardiographic assessment of the pressure gradient during bicycle ergometry in hypertrophic cardiomyopathy. Am J Cardiol 1992; 69: 1623–8.

25. Yock PG, Hatle L, Popp RL. Patterns and timing of Doppler-detected intracavitary and aortic flow in hypertrophic cardiomyopathy. J Am Coll Cardiol 1986; 8: 1047–58.

26. Kizilbash AM, Heinle SK, Grayburn PA. Spontaneous variability of left ventricular outflow tract gradient in hypertrophic obstructive cardiomyopathy. Circulation 1998; 97: 461–6.

27. Frans EE, Nanda NC, Patel V et al. Live three-dimensional transthoracic contrast echocardiographic assessment of apical hypertrophic cardiomyopathy. Echocardiography 2005; 22: 686–9.

28. Hubka M, Bolson EL, McDonald JA et al. Three-dimensional echocardiographic measurement of left and right ventricular mass and volume: in vitro validation. Int J Cardiovasc Imaging 2002; 18: 111–18.

29. Qin JX JM, Shiota T, Greenberg NL et al. New digital measurement methods for left ventricular volume using real-time three-dimensional echocardiography: comparison with electromagnetic flow method and magnetic resonance imaging. Eur J Echocardiogr 2000; 1: 96–104.

30. Schmidt MA, Ohazama CJ, Agyeman KO et al. Real-time three-dimensional echocardiography for measurement of left ventricular volumes. Am J Cardiol 1999; 84: 1434–9.

31. Qin JX, Jones M, Travaglini A et al. The accuracy of left ventricular mass determined by real-time three-dimensional echocardiography in chronic animal and clinical studies: a comparison with postmortem examination and magnetic resonance imaging. J Am Soc Echocardiogr 2005; 18: 1037–43.

32. Gopal AS, Schnellbaecher MJ, Shen Z et al. Freehand three-dimensional echocardiography for measurement of left ventricular mass: in vivo anatomic validation using explanted human hearts. J Am Coll Cardiol 1997; 30: 802–10.

33. Gopal AS, Keller AM, Shen Z et al. Three-dimensional echocardiography: in vitro and in vivo validation of left ventricular mass and comparison with conventional echocardiographic methods. J Am Coll Cardiol 1994; 24: 504–13.

34. Schmidt MA, Freidlin RZ, Ohazama CJ et al. Anatomic validation of a novel method for left ventricular volume and mass measurements with use of real-time 3-dimensional echocardiography. J Am Soc Echocardiogr 2001; 14: 1–10.

35. Sanada H, Shimizu M, Sugihara N et al. Increased left atrial chamber stiffness in hypertrophic cardiomyopathy. Br Heart J 1993; 69: 31–5.

36. Nagueh SF, Lakkis NM, Middleton KJ et al. Changes in left ventricular filling and left atrial function six months after nonsurgical septal reduction therapy for hypertrophic obstructive cardiomyopathy. J Am Coll Cardiol 1999; 34: 1123–8.

37. Bauer F, Shiota T, Qin JX, White RD, Thomas JD. Measurement of left atrial and ventricular volumes in real-time 3D echocardiography. Validation by nuclear magnetic resonance. Arch Mal Coeur Vaiss 2001; 94: 31–8.

38. Bauer F, Shiota T, White RD et al. Determinant of left atrial dilation in patients with hypertrophic cardiomyopathy: a real-time 3-dimensional echocardiographic study. J Am Soc Echocardiogr 2004; 17: 968–75.

39. Maron BJ. Hypertrophic cardiomyopathy [published erratum appears in Lancet 1997; 350(9087): 1330]. Lancet 1997; 350: 127–33.

40. Chikamori T, Counihan PJ, Doi YL et al. Mechanisms of exercise limitation in hypertrophic cardiomyopathy. J Am Coll Cardiol 1992; 19: 507–12.

41. Fananapazir L, McAreavey D. Therapeutic options in patients with obstructive hypertrophic cardiomyopathy and severe drug-refractory symptoms [editorial; comment]. J Am Coll Cardiol 1998; 31: 259–64.

42. Nishimura RA, Trusty JM, Hayes DL et al. Dual-chamber pacing for hypertrophic cardiomyopathy: a randomized, double-blind, crossover trial. J Am Coll Cardiol 1997; 29: 435–41.

43. Tascon JC, Albarran A, Hernandez F et al. Obstructive myocardiopathic hypertrophy and sequential atrioventricular stimulation. Immediate results and long term follow-up. Seven years experience. Rev Esp Cardiol 2000; 53: 1028–39.

44. Hess OM, Sigwart U. New treatment strategies for hypertrophic obstructive cardiomyopathy: alcohol ablation of the septum: the new gold standard? J Am Coll Cardiol 2004; 44: 2054–5.

45. Maron BJ, Dearani JA, Ommen SR et al. The case for surgery in obstructive hypertrophic cardiomyopathy. J Am Coll Cardiol 2004; 44: 2044–53.

46. Merrill WH, Friesinger GC, Graham TP Jr et al. Long-lasting improvement after septal myectomy for hypertrophic obstructive cardiomyopathy. Ann Thorac Surg 2000; 69: 1732–5.

47. Qin JX, Shiota T, Lever HM et al. Outcome of patients with hypertrophic obstructive cardiomyopathy after percutaneous transluminal septal myocardial ablation and septal myectomy surgery. J Am Coll Cardiol 2001; 38: 1994–2000.

48. Lakkis NM, Naguegh SF, Dunn JK, Killip D, Spencer WH. Nonsurgical septal reduction therapy for hypertrophic obstructive cardiomyopathy: one-year follow-up. J Am Coll Cardiol 2000; 36: 852–5.

49. Heric BLB, Miller DP, Rosenkranz ER, Lever HM, Cosgrove DM. Surgical management of hypertrophic obstructive cardiomyopathy. Early and late results. J Thorac Cardiovasc Surg 1995; 110: 195–206.

50. McCully RB, Nishimura RA, Tajik AJ, Schaff HV, Danielson GK. Extent of clinical improvement after surgical treatment of hypertrophic obstructive cardiomyopathy. Circulation 1996; 94: 467–71.

51. Salustri A, Kofflard MJ, Roelandt JR et al. Assessment of left ventricular outflow in hypertrophic cardiomyopathy using anyplane and paraplane analysis of three-dimensional echocardiography. Am J Cardiol 1996; 78: 462–8.

52. Franke A, Schondube FA, Kuhl HP et al. Quantitative assessment of the operative results after extended myectomy and surgical reconstruction of the subvalvular mitral apparatus in hypertrophic obstructive cardiomyopathy using dynamic three-dimensional transesophageal echocardiography. J Am Coll Cardiol 1998; 31: 1641–9.

53. Qin JX, Shiota T, Lever HM et al. Impact of left ventricular outflow tract area on systolic outflow velocity in hypertrophic cardiomyopathy: a real-time three-dimensional echocardiographic study. J Am Coll Cardiol 2002; 39: 308–14.

54. Sherrid MV, Chu CK, Delia E, Mogtader A, Dwyer EM Jr. An echocardiographic study of the fluid mechanics of obstruction in hypertrophic cardiomyopathy. J Am Coll Cardiol 1993; 22: 816–25.

55. Sitges M, Qin JX, Lever HM et al. Evaluation of left ventricular outflow tract area after septal reduction in obstructive hypertrophic cardiomyopathy: a real-time 3-dimensional echocardiographic study. Am Heart J 2005; 150: 852–8.

56. Nash PJ, Agler DA, Shin JH et al. Images in cardiovascular medicine. Epicardial real-time 3-dimensional echocardiography during septal myectomy for obstructive hypertrophic cardiomyopathy. Circulation 2003; 108: e54–5.

57. Willert JL, Shook D, D'Ambra MN. 3D transesophageal echocardiography: systolic anterior motion with hypertrophic obstructive cardiomyopathy. Anesth Analg 2006; 102: 1361–2.

58. Sitges MST, Tsujino H, Qin JX et al. Real-time three-dimensional color-Doppler evaluation of the flow convergence surface for quantification of mitral regurgitation. Circulation 2000; 102: II-629.

59. Irvine T, Derrick G, Morris D, Norton M, Kenny A. Three-dimensional echocardiographic reconstruction of mitral valve color Doppler flow events. Am J Cardiol 1999; 84: 1103–6, A10.

60. Shiota T, Sinclair B, Ishii M et al. Three-dimensional reconstruction of color Doppler flow convergence regions and regurgitant jets: an in vitro quantitative study. J Am Coll Cardiol 1996; 27: 1511–18.

61. De Simone R, Glombitza G, Vahl CF et al. Three-dimensional color Doppler: a clinical study in patients with mitral regurgitation. J Am Coll Cardiol 1999; 33: 1646–54.

13 Congenital Heart Disease

Philippe Acar

Three-dimensional (3D) echocardiography can provide an accurate description of various congenital heart diseases, as well as shunt and valve pathology. The introduction of real-time 3D echocardiography has led to its use in everyday clinical practice in the field of congenital heart disease. The 3D matrix probe enables the instantaneous acquisition of transthoracic volumes. Fetal 3D echocardiography is now available. Quantitative measurement of ventricular volumes could be obtained by 3D echocardiography. The utilization of the matrix probe should lead to routine use of 3D echocardiography, as for the 2D and Doppler methods. Its results should be decisive in many congenital cardiac lesions requiring surgery or interventional catheterization. This chapter is divided into three parts: (1) septal defects, (2) valve pathologies, and (3) fetal 3D echocardiography.

SEPTAL DEFECTS

Atrial septal defect

The selection of patients for transcatheter or surgical closure of a secundum atrial septal defect (ASD) requires accurate information regarding the anatomy of the defect, such as its maximal diameter and the amount of circumferential tissue rim. Two-dimensional (2D) echocardiography is insufficient to define criteria selection for ASD closure (Figures 13.1 and 13.2). Since the defect is visualized from multiple orthogonal planes, maximal ASD diameter is widely underestimated.[1] The transcatheter approach measures the stretched diameter but cannot be applied alone for patient selection since it does not provide information on the tissue rim.[2] 3D echocardiography allows unique *en face* views of the atrial septum (Figures 13.3 and 13.4). The success of ASD transcatheter closure is strongly related to the location and anatomy of the defect. Preselection of patients is a challenge for the pediatric cardiologist who needs an accurate and non-invasive method. Transthoracic 3D echocardiography is able to measure the maximal diameter and the tissue rim surrounding the ASD.[3,4] Two crucial parameters need to be determined: the tissue rim dimensions all around the defect to select patients for transcatheter closure, and the ASD maximal diameter in order to choose the appropriate size of the device.

Insufficient rim may result in migration of the ASD occluder. The minimal distance required before transcatheter closure depends on the device geometry. The Amplatzer septal occluder covers 7 mm all around the defect.[5] Since 2D echocardiography approaches the atrial septum from multiple orthogonal planes, it requires a mental 3D construction to comprehend the relation between the defect and the surrounding structures. Transthoracic 3D echocardiography allows surface imaging of the atrial septum. The ASD and the rims over 360° are simultaneously and directly imaged from the 3D echocardiography views.[6] We encountered the difficulties reported by Magni et al in visualizing the entire length of the posterior inferior rim by transesophageal 3D echocardiography.[7] Transthoracic 3D echocardiography depicted very well the inferior rims, as shown in Figures 13.5 and 13.6. According to the geometric profile of the Amplazter septal occluder, we ignored the superior anterior rim (distance from the aorta).

3D echocardiography can provide the atriotomy view on a beating heart and allows description of the ASD through the cardiac cycle.[8] One striking finding of 3D echocardiographic reconstructions was the great variability of the shape of the ASD (Figure 13.7). 3D transesophageal echocardiographic studies pointed out how the shape of the defect might alter the accuracy of diameter calculations by 2D echocardiography. In rounded ASDs, the 2D ultrasound beam may cut the defect in its maximal diameter, but this is no longer true in defects of complex shape. In patients with elongated oval-shaped

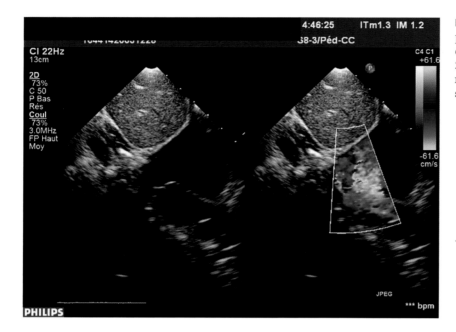

Figure 13.1 2D echocardiography in a patient with a secundum atrial septal defect. From the apical window, the 2D planes show enlargement of the right cavities with left to right atrial shunt.

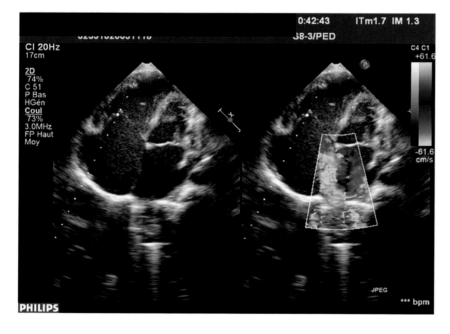

Figure 13.2 2D echocardiography in a patient with multiple atrial septal defects. From the subcostal window, multiple defect jets through the atrial septum are displayed.

defects, 2D echocardiography significantly underestimated the ASD maximal diameter. Moreover, the surface area of the ASD changed significantly during the cardiac cycle, with a maximum size in late ventricular systole and a minimum size in late left ventricular diastole. Such variation of the ASD area through the cardiac cycle increases the difficulty of determining the maximal diameter by selecting the right 2D frame. However, the balloon catheter method is still used as a reference to size the defect. The relation between the balloon stretched diameter and the ASD maximal diameter remains controversial. In patients with a floppy septum, we do realize that 3D echocardiography and balloon

sizing define different properties of an ASD. The 3D echocardiographic views can demonstrate the major axis, incorporating information about the shape of the ASD. Balloon sizing provides information about the degree of physical stretch, which cannot be predicted by 2D echocardiography.

By measuring ASD maximal diameter and tissue rims, 3D echocardiography helps to select patients for transcatheter ASD closure.[9] The size of the device should be fitted to the ASD size. Since the ASD area can be estimated from the 3D echocardiographic images it is unfortunate if the device area is not available for more accurate sizing. Transesophageal 2D echocardiography appears to

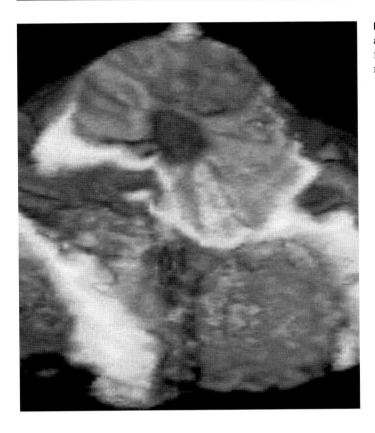

Figure 13.3 3D echocardiography of a secundum atrial septal defect. The atrial septal defect is viewed from the left atrium. The defect is single and has a round shape.

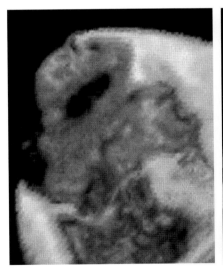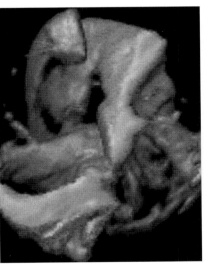

Figure 13.4 3D echocardiographic views of three atrial septal defects with complex shapes. Left (view from the right atrium): the defect is oval and single, far from a large right appendage anteriorly and from the tricuspid valve below. Right (view from the right atrium): the defects are multiple.

be adequate for assessment of the device placement. However, only a linear aspect of each disk may be simultaneously visualized of the atrial septum. Moreover, one cannot exactly determine where the 2D ultrasound beam insonates the disk, other than referencing the site to other anatomic landmarks. Hence, multiple orthogonal images are necessary to appreciate, albeit indirectly, the placement of the edges of each disk. 3D echocardiographic *en face* views could simultaneously and directly image the edges of either disk from the right or left atrial surface, almost exactly as the device appears in spatial reality. The geometric profile of the septal occluders can be described from the 3D views (Figure 13.8). McKendrick et al reported the use of real-time 3D echo to guide device closure of an ASD.[10] They concluded that this method was a feasible, safe, and effective alternative to the standard practice of transesophageal 2D echocardiography.

Ventricular septal defect

The ventricular septal defect (VSD) is the most common congenital heart malformation. Since 2D

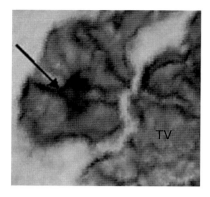

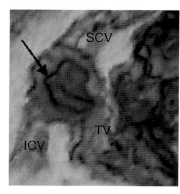

Figure 13.5 3D echocardiographic views from the right atrium. Left: central atrial septal defect (arrow). The large rims (> 4 mm) all around the defect allowed transcatheter closure with the Amplatzer septal occluder. Right: large atrial septal defect (arrow). The narrow rim (4 mm) from the tricuspid valve indicates surgical closure. TV, tricuspid valve; ICV, inferior caval vein; SCV, superior caval vein.

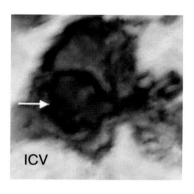

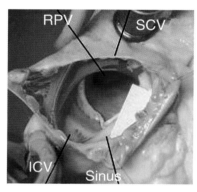

Figure 13.6 3D echocardiographic and surgical views from the right atrium. Left: large round atrial septal defect (arrow). The narrow rim (3 mm) from the inferior caval vein indicates surgical closure. Right: same patient. The surgical view confirms the deficient inferior posterior rim. RPV, right pulmonary vein; ICV, inferior caval vein; SCV, superior caval vein.

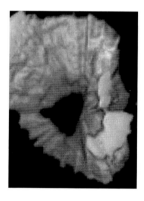

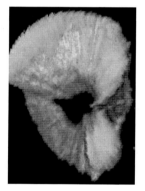

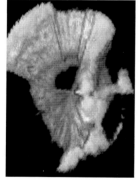

Figure 13.7 3D echocardiographic views of an atrial septal defect through the cardiac cycle. The temporal variations of the surface area of the septal defect viewed from the right atrium are illustrated in these three images of the same defect during late ventricular systole (left), mid-ventricular systole (middle), and end-ventricular diastole after atrial systole (right).

echocardiography approaches the ventricular septum from multiple orthogonal planes, it requires mental 3D construction to comprehend the relation between the defect and the surrounding structures (Figure 13.9). 3D echocardiography provide unique *en face* views of the ventricular septum (Figures 13.10 and 13.11). We reported the accuracy of 3D echocardiography in measuring muscular VSDs compared to surgery.[11] However, 3D echocardiography was limited with off-line reconstructions and variable image quality. The introduction of the 3D matrix-array probe allows real-time 3D rendering with higher resolution. Cheng et al reported a real-time 3D echocardiography study in assessing VSD.[12] They found an excellent correlation in measurement of the size

of VSDs by 3D echocardiography compared to surgery.

Transcatheter closure of perimembranous VSDs has been attempted as an alternative approach to surgery.[13] The specific device has to be positioned very closely to the aortic and tricuspid valve (Figures 13.12 and 13.13). The 3D *en face* views allow better comprehension of the VSD and its relation to adjacent structures. The location of the defect in the membranous septum explains the risk for the valves.[14] The perimembranous VSD is located in the outlet portion of the left ventricle immediately beneath the aortic valve. The presence of a 2 mm or more rim of tissue between the defect and the aortic valve is generally required for device closure of perimembranous VSDs. The septal leaflet

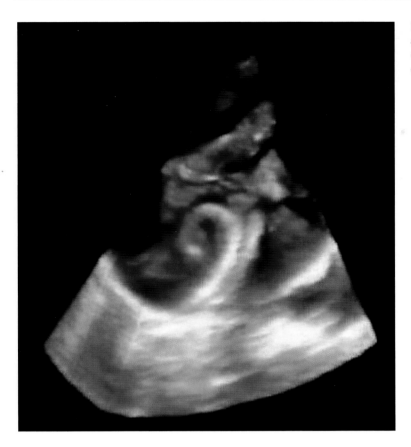

Figure 13.8 3D echocardiography of an atrial septal occluder. The Amplatzer septal occluder viewed from the right atrium has a concave shape in the right atrial cavity.

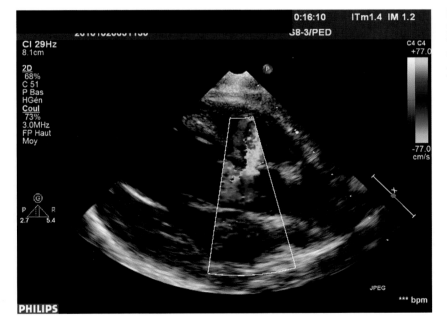

Figure 13.9 2D echocardiography in a patient with a ventricular septal defect. The perimembranous septal defect with a left to right shunt is seen from a parasternal long-axis view.

of the tricuspid valve is in continuity with the aortic leaflets. Moreover, extra septal leaflet tissue can partially occlude the defect. Such a complicated relation between the perimembranous VSD and the aortic and tricuspid leaflets could be displayed by 3D views from the left and the right side.[15] The Amplatzer membranous VSD occluder has a specific profile consisting of two parallel disks with minimal subaortic rim (Figure 13.14).

VALVE PATHOLOGIES

Ebstein malformation

Ebstein malformation is a rare congenital heart disease. Patients with Ebstein anomaly have a wide spectrum of anatomic abnormalities. The predictors of outcome depend on the severity of the tricuspid valve malformation.[16,17] A precise

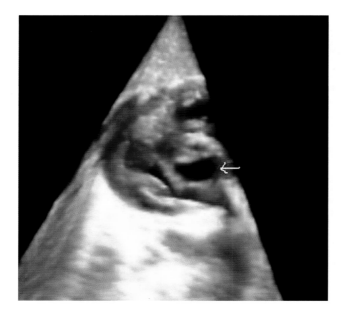

Figure 13.10   3D echocardiography of a perimembranous ventricular septal defect. The defect (arrow) viewed from the left ventricle has an oval shape. The maximal diameter of the defect could be appreciated accurately.

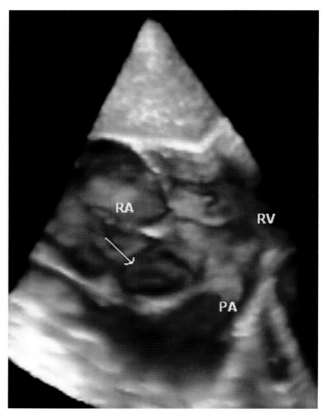

Figure 13.12   3D echocardiography of a perimembranous ventricular septal defect. The defect (arrow) is viewed from the right side. The closed relation between the perimembranous ventricular septal defect and the septal leaflet of the tricuspid valve is clearly displayed. RA, right atrium; RV, right ventricle; PA, pulmonary artery.

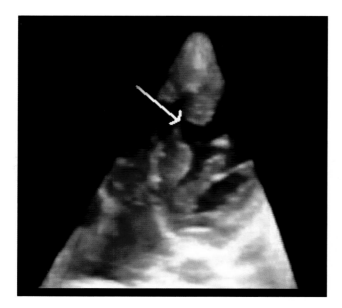

Figure 13.11   3D echocardiography of a muscular ventricular septal defect. The defect (arrow) viewed from the right ventricle is located in the mid-muscular septum.

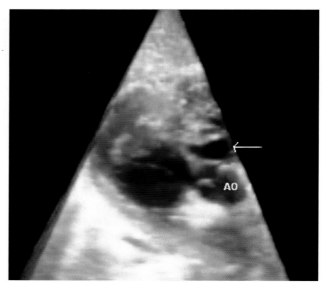

Figure 13.13   3D echocardiography of a perimembranous ventricular septal defect. The defect (arrow) is viewed from the left ventricle. The tiny rim between the perimembranous ventricular septal defect and the aortic leaflets (AO) requires a specific profile of the device. The Amplatzer membranous VSD occluder has an eccentric left disk with minimal subaortic rim.

description of the tricuspid anatomy by conventional 2D echocardiography remains difficult. 3D echocardiography offers surface rendering views of the leaflet surface.[18,19] Ebstein anomaly of the tricuspid valve consists of various degrees of inferior displacement of the proximal attachments of the septal leaflet. Since the apical 4-chamber plane provides good visualization of the septal leaflet, 2D echocardiography allows the initial diagnosis

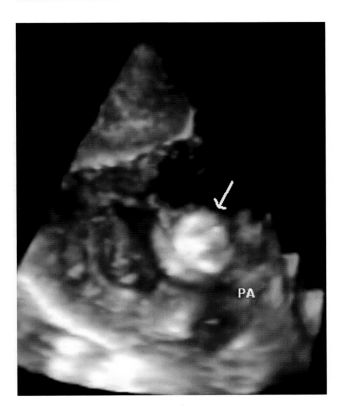

Figure 13.14 3D echocardiography of a ventricular septal occluder. The Amplatzer perimembranous ventricular septal defect occluder is viewed from the right side. The right disk (arrow) is well positioned close to the septum and far from the pulmonary artery valve (PA).

of Ebstein anomaly (Figures 13.15 and 13.16). However, downward displacement could involve the anterior and posterior leaflets of the tricuspid valve. A precise description of the tricuspid valve anatomy is difficult from the 2D planes only. The surface of the tricuspid leaflets as well as the commissures could be rendered by 3D echocardiography (Figures 13.17 and 13.18). 3D echocardiography can offer new and unique views to evaluate the potential and efficiency of surgical valve repair (Figure 13.19).

Bicuspid aortic valve

Espinola-Zavaleta et al verified the echocardiographic characteristics of the bicuspid aortic valve using 3D transesophageal echocardiography by comparing the findings with anatomic examination of autopsy specimens from carriers of this condition.[20] There was a clear correspondence between anatomic and echocardiographic findings, which led to the conclusion that 3D echocardiography is a technique that reliably defines the morphologic details of the bicuspid aortic valve with the precision of anatomo-pathologic examination (Figure 13.20). We reported the effect of balloon dilatation on aortic stenosis assessed by 3D echocardiography. A 10-year-old boy with a bicuspid

valve treated by surgical valvulotomy when he was 6 months old underwent balloon dilatation of recurrent aortic stenosis.[21] The anatomy of the aortic valve and effects of the balloon dilatation were clearly visualized on the 3D views (Figure 13.21).

Cleft mitral valve

Mitral regurgitation is a major cause of late morbidity after surgical repair of atrioventricular septal defect. Past studies have indicated that up to 40% of the patients ultimately require reoperation. Detailed preoperative description of the valve malformation is essential in clinical decision-making, whether the valve is amenable for repair or an artificial valve is unavoidable. Studies reported that 3D echocardiography provides a better understanding of the dynamic morphology of the mitral valve and its relation with the surrounding structures in patients after atrioventricular septal defect repair compared to 2D echocardiography.[22–24] With the 3D views, the mitral valve can be displayed as the anatomic diagrams of the atrioventricular valve malformations. The variability in morphology of the superior and inferior bridging leaflet that can be visualized in 3D, together with the hemodynamic information of the 2D echocardiography leads to a better understanding of the complex anatomy (Figures 13.22–13.24).

FETAL 3D ECHOCARDIOGRAPHY

Fetal echocardiography has been used to screen, diagnose, monitor, and treat congenital heart defects and rhythm abnormalities. Conventional real-time echocardiography can only display 2D structural images of the intricate 3D fetal heart. 3D echocardiography has been shown to enhance the diagnosis of congenital heart disease in children. However, because of the difficulty in obtaining a fetal electrocardiogram to gate the heart, the development of fetal 3D echocardiography has been limited. With the advent of a new transthoracic matrix-array probe that allows real-time 3D data acquisition and image rendering, many of the above limitations could be circumvented. Real-time 3D echocardiography is a recent technique which allows direct visualization without ECG gating.[25] The cardiac matrix probe offers a new mode of 3D fetal echocardiography rendering and biplane imaging (Figures 13.25 and 13.26).

CONCLUSIONS

3D echocardiography can provide unique *en face* views of the heart valves and septa that are not obtainable with conventional 2D transthoracic and transesophageal echocardiography. The recent

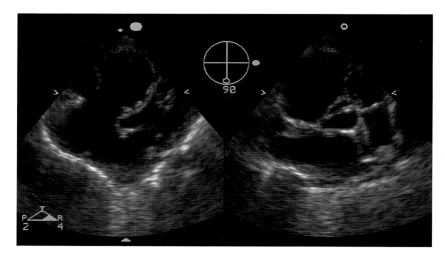

Figure 13.15 Biplane echocardiography in a neonate with severe Ebstein anomaly. The 4-chamber plane (left) shows attachment of the septal and anterior leaflets with an enlarged right atrium. The orthogonal plane (right) depicts the apical coaptation of the tricuspid valve. Right ventricle volume was reduced to the outflow tract. The pulmonary valve was closed in systole, creating a functional atresia.

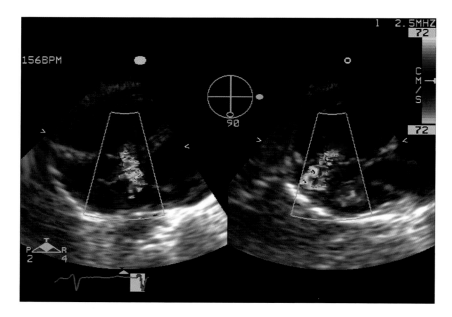

Figure 13.16 Biplane echocardiography in a 6-year-old female with Ebstein anomaly. Color Doppler was added to the biplane imaging to assess extension and severity of tricuspid regurgitation. Tricuspid regurgitation had an origin near the interventricular septum (left) with a mild extension into the right atrium (right).

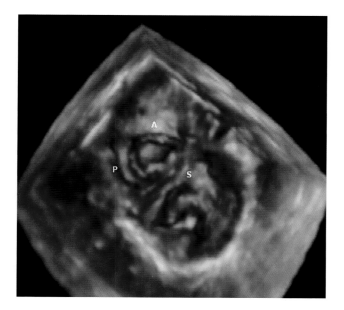

Figure 13.17 3D echocardiography in an infant with moderate Ebstein anomaly. The tricuspid valve was viewed from the right ventricle. The three leaflets with the commissures were visualized from below. Only the septal (S) leaflet had abnormal attachment to the ventricular septum. Anterior (A) and posterior (P) leaflets had normal coaptation.

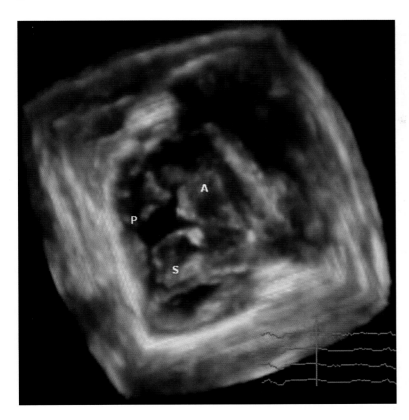

Figure 13.18 3D echocardiography in an adolescent with severe Ebstein anomaly. The tricuspid valve was viewed from below. Because of a restrictive motion and reduced functional surface, the posterior leaflet did not coapt with the septal (S) leaflet. The posterior (P) commissure appeared as a huge hole compared to the continent anterior (A) and septal commissures.

A   B   C

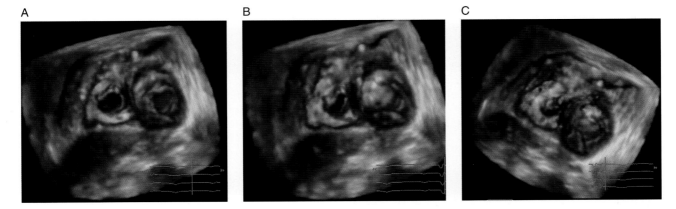

Figure 13.19 3D echocardiography in a 12-year-old boy after Ebstein repair. The tricuspid and mitral valves were viewed from below: (A) early diastole (mitral and tricuspid valves opened); (B) end-diastole (mitral valve closed and tricuspid valve opened); (C) systole (mitral and tricuspid valves closed). The surgically enlarged anterior leaflet was the only mobile leaflet. The tricuspid valve repair created a functional monocusp with trivial regurgitation without stenosis.

introduction of the transthoracic and transesophageal 3D matrix-array probes allow real-time 3D rendering. Thus, it should lead to routine usage of 3D echocardiography as with the 2D and Doppler methods. 3D echocardiology should add considerable value to decision-making in many congenital cardiac lesions requiring surgery or interventional catheterization.

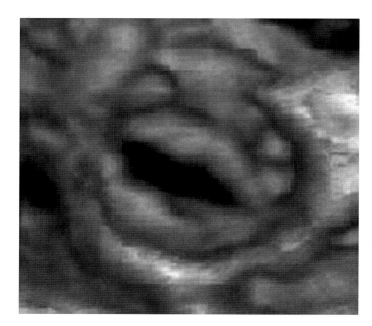

Figure 13.20 3D echocardiography in an infant with a bicuspid aortic valve. The aortic valve is viewed from above. The edges and the surface of the leaflets are thickened.

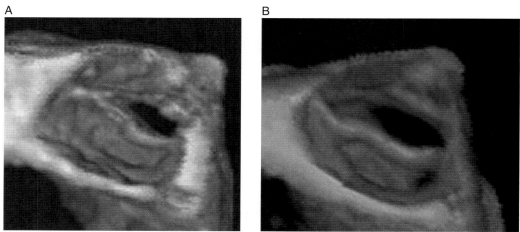

A   B

Figure 13.21 3D echocardiography before and after balloon dilatation. The bicuspid aortic valve is viewed from the aorta in systole. (A) Before dilatation, the fusion of the anterior commissure associated with the thickness of the leaflet edges makes the valve stenotic. The posterior commissure is free. Opening surface of valve is 0.7 cm². (B) After dilatation, the anterior commissure is clearly opened after balloon inflation. Opening surface is now 1.2 cm².

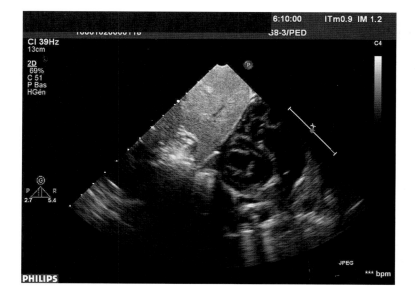

Figure 13.22 2D echocardiography in a patient with a cleft mitral valve. From the subcostal window, the cleft divides the anterior mitral valve into superior and inferior leaflets.

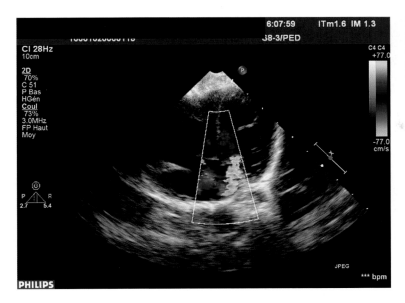

Figure 13.23 2D echocardiography in a patient with mitral regurgitation. From the apical window, the mitral regurgitation originates through the cleft of the anterior mitral valve.

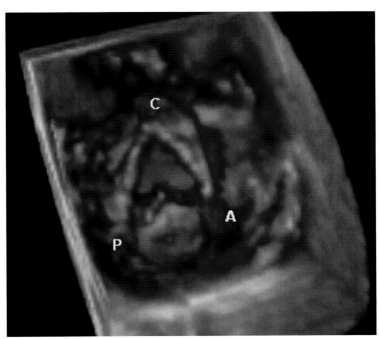

Figure 13.24 3D echocardiography in a 6-year-old female with an isolated cleft mitral valve. The valve is viewed from below. The anterior mitral valve is divided into two equivalent leaflets by a cleft (C). The anterior (A) and posterior (P) commissures as well as the papillary muscles underneath are well seen delineating the posterior mitral valve.

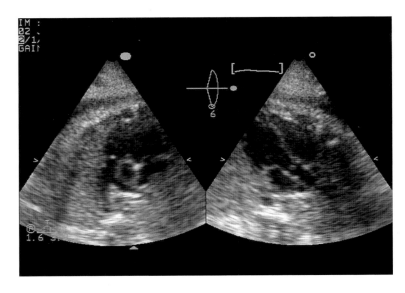

Figure 13.25 Biplane echocardiography of a normal fetal heart. The matrix transducer allows simultaneous display of two planes without moving the transducer. By a rotational and lateral tilt to 6°, the left and right ventricular outflow chambers are obtained simultaneously. The pulmonary bifurcation is clearly seen as well as the mitro-aortic continuity.

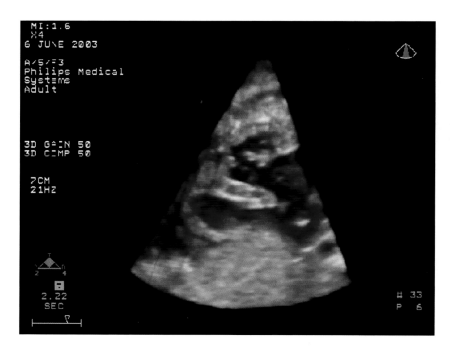

Figure 13.26 3D echocardiography of a normal fetal heart. Both left and right ventricles have a volume rendering. By cropping the pyramid, intracardiac views of the ventricle were obtained. The right ventricle was clearly recognizable by the trabeculations compared to the smooth left ventricle.

REFERENCES

1. Mehta R, Helmcke F, Nanda NC et al. Uses and limitations of transthoracic echocardiography in the assessment of atrial septal defect in adults. Am J Cardiol 1991; 67: 288–94.

2. Rao PS, Langhough R, Beekman RH, Lloyd TR, Sideris EB. Echocardiographic estimation of balloon-stretched diameter of secundum atrial septal defect for transcatheter occlusion. Am Heart J 1992; 124: 172–5.

3. Marx GR, Fulton DR, Pandian NG et al. Delineation of site, relative size and dynamic geometry of atrial septal defect by real-time three-dimensional echocardiography. J Am Coll Cardiol 1995; 25: 482–90.

4. Acar P, Saliba Z, Bonhoeffer P et al. Influence of atrial septal defect anatomy in patient selection and assessment of closure by the CardioSEAL device: a three-dimensional transesophageal echocardiography. Eur Heart J 2000; 21: 573–81.

5. Acar P, Saliba Z, Bonhoeffer P et al. Assessment of the geometric profile of the Amplatzer and Cardioseal occluders by three-dimensional echocardiography. Heart 2001; 85: 451–3.

6. Hellenbrand WE, Fahey JT, McFowan FX et al. Transesophageal echocardiographic guidance of transcatheter closure of atrial septal defect. Am J Cardiol 1990; 66: 207–13.

7. Magni G, Hijazi Z, Pandian NG et al. Two- and three-dimensional transesophageal echocardiography in patient selection and assessment of atrial septal defect closure by the new DAS-Angel wings device. Circulation 1997; 96: 1722–8.

8. Franke A, Kühl HP, Rulands D et al. Quantitative analysis of the morphology of secundum-type atrial septal defects and their dynamic change using transesophageal three-dimensional echocardiography. Circulation 1997; 96(Suppl II): II-323–7.

9. Acar P, Dulac Y, Roux D et al. Comparison of tranthoracic and transesophageal three-dimensional echocardiography for assessment of atrial septal defect diameter in children. Am J Cardiol 2003; 91: 500–2.

10. McKendrick R, Owada CY. Real-time 3D echocardiography-guided transcatheter device closure of atrial septal defects. Cathet Cardiovasc Interven 2005; 65: 442–6.

11. Acar P, Abdel-Massih T, Douste-Blazy MY et al. Assessment of muscular ventricular septal defect closure by transcatheter or surgical approach: a three-dimensional echocardiographic study. Eur J Echocardiography 2002; 3: 185–91.

12. Cheng TO, Xie MX, Wang XF et al. Real-time 3-dimensional echocardiography in assessing atrial and ventricular septal defects: an echocardiographic–surgical correlative study. Am Heart J 2004; 148: 1091–5.

13. Fu YC, Bass J, Amin Z, Radtke W et al. Transcatheter closure of perimembranous ventricular septal defects using the new Amplatzer membranous VSD occluder. J Am Coll Cardiol 2006; 47: 319–25.

14. Ho SY, McCarthy KP, Rigby ML. Morphology of perimembranous ventricular septal defects: implications for transcatheter device closure. J Interven Cardiol 2004; 17: 99–108.

15. Acar P, Abadir S, Aggoun Y. Transcatheter closure of perimembranous ventricular septal defects with Amplatzer occluder assessed by real-time 3D echocardiography. Eur J Echocardiography 2006 in press.

16. Celermajer DS, Bull C, Till JA et al. Ebstein's anomaly: presentation and outcome from fetus to adult. J Am Coll Cardiol 1994; 23: 170–6.

17. Gussenhoven EJ, Stewart PA, Becker AE et al. 'Offsetting' of the septal tricuspid leaflet in normal hearts and in hearts with Ebstein's anomaly. Anatomic and echographic correlation. Am J Cardiol 1984; 54: 172–6.

18. Acar P, Abadir S, Taktak A et al. Ebstein's anomaly assessed by real-time three-dimensional echocardiography. Ann Thorac Surg 2006 in press.

19. Ahmed S, Nanda NC, Nekkanti R et al. Transesophageal three-dimensional echocardiographic demonstration of Ebstein's anomaly. Echocardiography 2003; 20: 305–7.

20. Espinola-Zavaleta N, Muñoz-Castellanos L, Attié F et al. Anatomic three-dimensional echocardiographic correlation of bicuspid aortic valve. J Am Soc Echocardiogr 2003; 16: 46–53.

21. Acar P, Aggoun Y, Saliba Z et al. Effect of balloon dilatation on aortic stenosis assessed by three-dimensional echocardiographic reconstruction. Circulation 1999; 99: 2598–9.

22. Acar P, Laskari C, Rhodes J et al. Determinants of mitral regurgitation after atrioventricular septal defect surgery: a three-dimensional echocardiographic study. Am J Cardiol 1999; 83: 745–9.

23. van den Bosch AE, van Dijk VF, McGhie JS et al. Real-time transthoracic three-dimensional echocardiography provides additional information of left-sided AV valve morphology after AVSD repair. Int J Cardiol 2006; 106: 360–4.

24. Abadir S, Dulac Y, Taktak A et al. Cleft mitral valve assessed by transthoracic real-time 3D echocardiography. Heart 2005; 91: 1632.

25. Acar P, Dulac Y, Taktak A et al. Real time three-dimensional fetal echocardiography using cardiac matrix probe. Prenatal Diagn 2005; 25: 370–5.

14 Strain Echocardiography

Asbjørn Stoylen

DEFINITIONS

Strain rate imaging (SRI) is an imaging method for deformation. Although the method was originally based on tissue Doppler imaging (TDI),[1] deformation imaging now has the possibility of utilizing other methods, such as speckle tracking,[2,3] or a combination of both. Other methods may become feasible in the future.[4] The basic concept, however, is not dependent on the method of deriving the velocity information, and the clinical use of the method will be similar.

Strain and strain rate

Strain simply means deformation. The original definition of strain that is still used clinically is relative change in length:

$$\varepsilon = \frac{L - L_0}{L_0}$$

Where L_0 is the original length and L is the length after deformation. This entity is dimensionless, and is usually expressed in percent. From the formula, shortening is negative, lengthening is positive strain, a cause of much linguistic confusion, as strain rate today is mostly concerned about longitudinal deformation, where the systolic contraction is longitudinal shortening, i.e. negative, but where the main interest is the magnitude of contraction.

The typical longitudinal strain in a healthy heart is in the order of -15 to -25%. Strain rate is the rate of change in strain, i.e. the change in strain per time unit:

$$SR = \frac{d\varepsilon}{dt}$$

It can be shown that this temporal derivative of strain can be measured as the spatial derivative of velocity, i.e. the change in velocity per length unit,

and can be expressed simply as the velocity gradient along or across the wall:

$$SR = \frac{v_2 - v_1}{D}$$

where v_1 and v_2 are two velocities measured at different points in the wall, and D is the offset distance between the two points. In fact this concept can be used for assessing strain rate in a semiquantitative way by simply looking at the separation of velocity curves (Figure 14.1).

The unit of strain rate is 1/s, usually written s^{-1}. In a healthy heart, the peak systolic strain rate is typically in the range of -1 to $-1.4\ s^{-1}$. Unlike velocities, the motion due to the contraction of remote segments as well as due to the overall motion of the heart is subtracted.

This simplified algorithm is in most systems substituted with a linear regression method along the offset distance. This means that the strain rate is equivalent to the velocity gradient described earlier,[5,6] however, the velocity gradient being applied basically to the transmural direction, while strain rate imaging has been applied to the longitudinal deformation.

Given the velocity data, displacement can be obtained by temporal integration of velocity, strain rate by spatial derivation of velocity (velocity difference per length unit), and strain can be obtained by temporal integration of strain rate (Figure 14.2).

Strain and strain rate show regional deformation only, and unlike velocity and displacement, the curves can be interpreted independently of the location in the myocardium.

Strain rate and strain have different physiologic significances. End-systolic strain measures the total amount of systolic deformation, and is dependent on load, ejection time, etc. It has been shown to correlate most closely with stroke volume and ejection fraction (EF),[7,8] while peak systolic strain rate correlates most closely with contractility.[8,9]

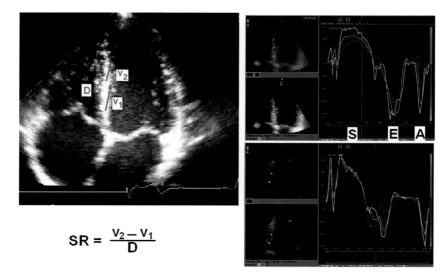

$$SR = \frac{V_2 - V_1}{D}$$

Figure 14.1 Strain as velocity gradient. Left: as the apex is relatively stationary, and the base is moving towards the apex during systole, the velocities are decreasing from the base to the apex. By measuring the velocity at two points, the velocity gradient can be estimated, giving strain rate. Right: the top panel shows the normal decreasing tissue velocities from base to apex. There are positive velocities during systole (S), as the myocardium moves towards the apex, and negative velocities as the myocardium moves away from the apex during early relaxation (E) and atrial systole (A). The difference between the curves is a direct visualization of the strain rate of the segment between the corresponding points. The bottom panel is from a patient with an extensive inferior infarction. All three velocity curves overlap. This means that there is no velocity difference between the three points, i.e. the whole wall is moving as a stiff plate, showing no deformation in the segments between the points. This is equivalent to the strain rate between the points being zero. The motion of the wall is solely due to contraction of the myocardium apical to the red point, the infracted area being tethered to this.

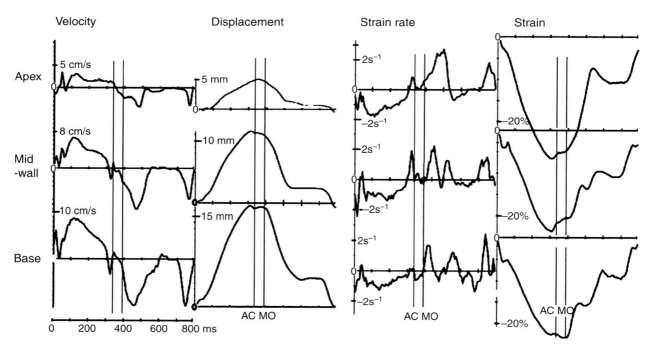

Figure 14.2 Typical curves from a normal subject. Left: velocities. Notice the decreasing velocities from base to apex. The second column from the left shows the displacement curves obtained by integrating the velocity curves. Notice that there is decreasing displacement from base to apex. The third column shows strain rate. The strain rate is negative during systole, as there is shortening, and positive during the diastolic lenthening. There are no significant differences between the levels in peak systolic strain rate. The right column shows the strain obtained by integrating the strain rate. The strain is negative during the whole heart cycle, increasingly so during systole, decreasingly during diastole.

Strain in three dimensions

Deformation in the heart muscle does not occur in only the longitudinal direction, as illustrated in Figure 14.3. The heart muscle being incompressible, in systole longitudinal and circumferential shortening has to be balanced by transmural thickening. So far the strains in each direction have to be measured sequentially.

Tissue Doppler can only measure thickening in the anteroseptal and inferolateral wall, where the beam is transverse to the wall, as the transmural velocity gradient,[5] although attempts at angle correction have been made,[6] and (at best) circumferential shortening where the beam is tangential to the wall in the short-axis direction.

Speckle tracking across the wall[3] can in principle measure deformation in two directions simultaneously, longitudinal and transmural in the apical direction and transmural and circumferential in the short-axis views.[3,10,11]

However, limitations in the lateral tracking may render the method of limited value.[12] Finally, the added value of measuring strain in more than one direction has to be documented, as the deformations in the three directions are interrelated.

Another approach to three-dimensional (3D) strain rate imaging is the 3D rendering of longitudinal strain and strain rate data,[13] as shown in Figure 14.4. This figure is reconstructed from three standard apical lanes by drawing a curved M-mode along the wall and processed using both strain rate data and the curvature information, as well as interpolation between the planes and cycles in time. Unlike other parametric imaging methods, this shows the true area of dyssynergy, and may be used quantitatively in the future.

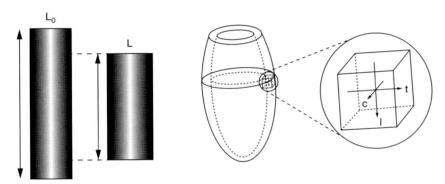

Figure 14.3 Strain in three dimensions. A solid object does not deform in one direction only, and if the body is incompressible, like heart muscle, the object has to deform in more than one direction simultaneously, so that the volume is preserved, as illustrated by the cylinder at the left. In the heart muscle (right), the three directions usually considered are longitudinal (l), transmural (t) and circumferential (c).

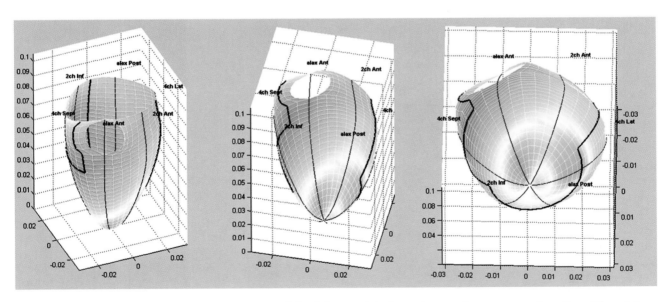

Figure 14.4 Three-dimensional reconstruction of the left ventricle in early systole as a curved surface. The picture shows an apical infarction with early systolic stretching in the infarct area (blue) as opposed to the normally contracting myocardium in the rest of the ventricle (yellow). The dataset is fully 3D, and can be rotated in space as shown by the display that is rotated from the anterior to the apical aspect.

PARAMETRIC IMAGING

Parametric imaging means displaying numeric data as a color map. It reduces the data to semiquantitative information for visual assessment, analogous to, for instance, wall motion score. Color flow is a typical example, but tissue velocities have been displayed the same way, and also strain rate and strain. 3D reconstruction as described above, curved M-mode, and bull's eye display are all parametric display modes. The curved anatomic M-mode[14] is an M-mode that is drawn within the myocardial wall, displaying strain rate as a color display in a time–strain rate plot, as shown in Figure 14.5. This gives semiquantitative strain rate information, but quantitative time–depth information.

As strain rate shifts from negative (shortening) to positive (lengthening) during the heart cycle (see Figure 14.2), the change in direction is more easily shown by color coding. Strain remains negative during the heart cycle, except in the case of initial stretching, and is thus less suited to parametric images. Analyzing traces, however, may be easier with strain, due to the noise reduction.

METHODS

Tissue Doppler

From the beginning, strain rate was measured by tissue Doppler by processing the velocity gradient.[1,5] The velocity gradient can then only be measured along each ultrasound beam. This limits the validity of the measurements; if the longitudinal deformation direction has an angle deviation from the ultrasound beam, not only will the reduced angle give reduced velocity measurements due to the cosine factor, but the beam will also incorporate a measure of transmural thickening, also detracting from the strain and strain rate values measured,[15] as seen in Figure 14.6. The angle problem is greatest if the images are poorly aligned (Figure 14.6(A)) and in the extreme apex and sometimes in the base (Figure 14.6(B)).

The advantage of tissue Doppler is its high frame rate, giving information of rapid phases in the heart cycle.

Speckle tracking

The method of speckle tracking is based on the unique pattern generated by the interference pattern from the scatterers and the reflected ultrasound.[16] The speckles are relatively stable during the heart cycle. This means that the motion can be tracked independently of the beam direction across the scan plane, and gives a true longitudinal strain rate. The method is thus angle independent. The limitation is the frame rate, giving a low temporal resolution. In addition, too low a frame rate or too high a heart rate may give changes from frame to frame that may reduce the quality of tracking.

LIMITATIONS

The main limitations of strain rate imaging, in addition to the angle limitation inherent in tissue

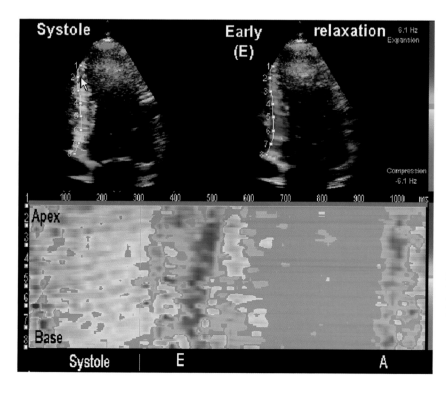

Figure 14.5 Curved anatomic M-mode (CAMM). The upper half shows two frames from systole and early diastole. In systole there is shortening, negative strain rate, coded as yellow. In early diastole there is lengthening, positive strain, coded in blue. A curved line is drawn manually within the septum from apex to base, and is shown on the 2D images. Below is the M-mode along this line. The numbers shown to the left are the same as in the 2D images, and are for orientation only. The time scale is on top of the M-mode. Systole is shown as a wide orange bar, early diastole (E) is shown in blue, and it can be seen that the elongation propagates from the base to the apex. Elongation during atrial systole (A) is also shown as an elongation wave. Diastasis with no deformation is green.

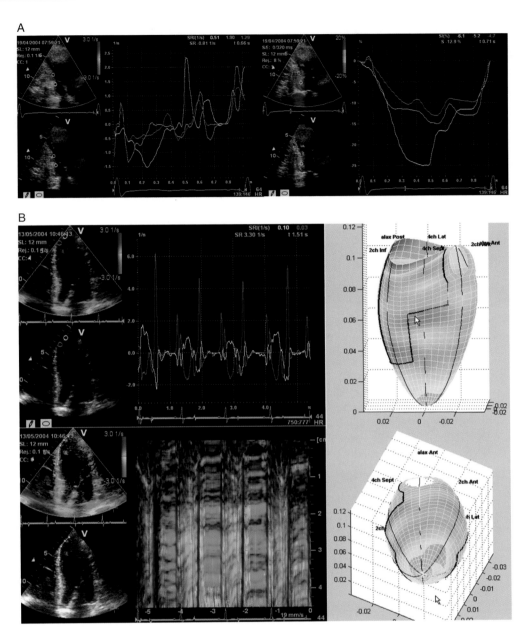

Figure 14.6 Angle dependence. (A) Two-chamber view that is poorly aligned. The apical half of the inferior wall is seen at an angle, so the transverse thickening detracts from the longitudinal shortening. There are normal strain rate and strain in the base (yellow traces), reduced strain rate and strain in the apical segment (red traces). In between there is a variation through the cycle, resulting in a normal strain rate early, but reduced strain rate late, resulting in a reduced overall strain. This illustrates the difference between the two parameters, as peak strain rate will remain normal although the rest of the curve is subject to artefacts. (B) Angle effects in the apex of a normal subject in a well-aligned image. To the left are the traces and the curved M-mode. There is normal strain rate in the septum, also in the basal part of the apical segment (red trace, red systolic bars). In the extreme apex there is angle effect, giving inverted strain values (thickening) seen in the yellow trace and in the blue color on top of the systolic bars in the M-mode. To the right is a 3D reconstruction from the same subject, showing the area affected to be fairly small.

Doppler as described above, are related to image quality.[14] The most important limitations are reverberations and drop outs, as shown in Figures 14.7 and 14.8. We have previously shown that about 85% of patients have segments that have to be discarded due to poor image quality and, hence, poor data.[17,18] So far, there are few studies addressing the feasibility of segments in terms of speckle tracking, but it seems, not surprisingly, to be of the same order.[10,11,17]

When using strain rate imaging, the most important point is to rigidly exclude areas with poor

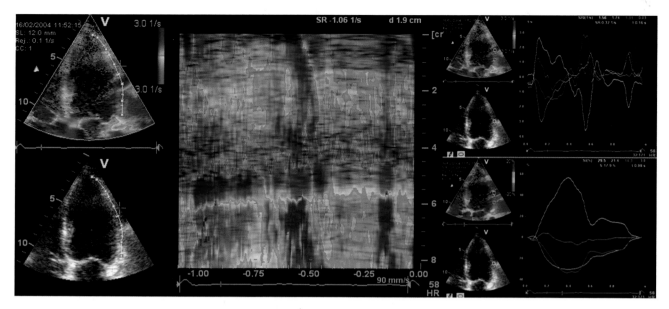

Figure 14.7 Stationary reverberation. The reverberation results in an echo that is motionless. This can be seen as the heavy white band in the lateral wall. In the CAMM, the reverberation is a thick band of inverted color, blue in systole and orange in diastole. The location, corresponding to no known coronary territory, the horizontal course, not following the myocardial motion, and the rapid shift from deep colors at the borders makes it easy to identify. The strain rate and strain traces are not so evidently artificial, however. Below the reverberation is an overestimation of the strain rate (cyan trace), above is an inverted strain rate and strain curve (yellow traces). Both curves, however, are artificial, and due to either v_1 or v_2 in the algorithm being zero. In between there are in between values (green and red), where the green shows initial stretching and reduced strain, while the red shows normal strain and strain rate, both simply due to the interpolation between the yellow and cyan traces.

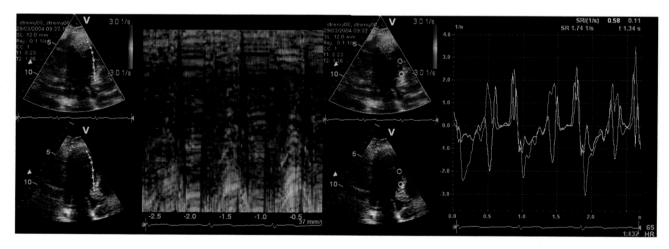

Figure 14.8 Drop out. There is a drop out in the apical anterior septum. In the apex there are no data and, hence, no strain rate, as seen in the M-mode. Below is an area of overestimated strain rate (red), cyan trace, due to the algorithm subtracting normal velocities from zero velocities in the dropout area.

image quality, and not try to eke out meaningful information, as this may lead to erroneous conclusions based on artefacts (Figures 14.7 and 14.8).

CLINICAL USE

The main use of strain rate imaging is in evaluating regional systolic function. For global function, the method can yield global parameters such as global strain[19] or global peak strain rate.[20] However, it remains to be shown that these methods give a better diagnostic accuracy than longitudinal shortening[21] or annular velocity,[22] respectively, the latter being less processed and, hence, more robust.

For diastolic function, the annular velocities are still the main method, as the diastolic pattern of strain rate is complex.[23] Thus the main use is in regional heterogeneity of function, i.e. in ischemic heart disease, to some extent in cardiomyopathies, and it may have a use in resynchronization therapy.

In order to use strain rate imaging, it should be emphasized that the information is additional to the rest of the information. Isolated strain rate data are less useful.[18]

The parametric images are more robust, identifying not only areas of poor image quality, but giving information through the time–depth distribution of the colors (Figure 14.9). In addition, the color gives a semiquantitative wall motion score, shown to be comparable to the wall motion score from 2D echocardiography,[24,25] as shown in Figure 14.10.

For full quantitative analysis, the traces are available. The quantitative traces are most easily evaluated in strain, as the temporal integration will give a smoothing of the curves. However, newer software has implemented smoothing in strain rate that results in more readable strain rate curves as well (Figure 14.11). Both sets of curves

show the same effect; findings may vary from total stretching during the whole systole, via initial stretching and subsequent hypokinesia to mild hypokinesia. Post-systolic shortening is a frequent finding in acute infarction as well as ischemia;[26] it tends to decrease with time after the infarction.[27] It is shown to be a marker of ischemia, but there is still discussion of whether it is also a viability marker in the acute phase (Figure 14.12). The post-systolic strain should not exceed 3% of the total strain in order to be within normal range. Peak systolic strain should be lower than -1 s^{-1}, end-systolic strain lower than -15%.

The presence of post-systolic shortening has also been shown to be a marker of ischemia in stress echo[28] (Figure 14.13), although peak-systolic strain rate at peak stress may be as useful.[29] The cut off at peak stress should be between -1.2 and 1.3. The timing of onset of shortening and post systolic shortening is also very well suited to parametric imaging, as shown in Figure 14.14.[28]

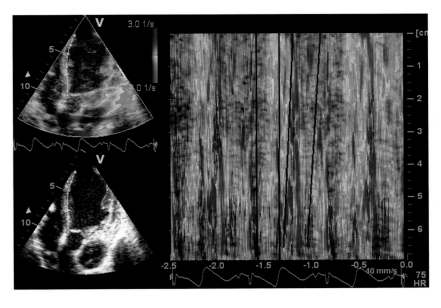

Figure 14.9 Curved M-mode through an area of shadowy reverberations that affects the strain rate despite fairly good gray scale visibility. This finding excludes any kind of quantitative analysis, but even so, the phases and timing can be discerned as broken bands, indicated by the black lines in the second cycle.

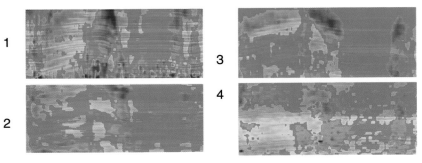

Figure 14.10 Wall motion score (WMS) by color SRI. All panels show curved M-modes of one heart cycle, apex on top, base at the bottom. WMS numbers are shown at each panel. 1: Normal systolic function. 2: Hypokinesia in the basal part, there is late onset and reduced magnitude (as seen by the spotted pattern due to noise) of the shortening (orange). In addition there is orange color after the end of systole; post-systolic shortening indicative of acute ischemia. 3: Akinesia. There is no systolic shortening in the basal half at all. In addition, there is marked post-systolic shortening, another pathologic finding. 4: Dyskinesia. There is stretching of the apex, as indicated by the blue color in systole. That this is not an artefact is substantiated by the post-systolic shortening seen after end-systole.

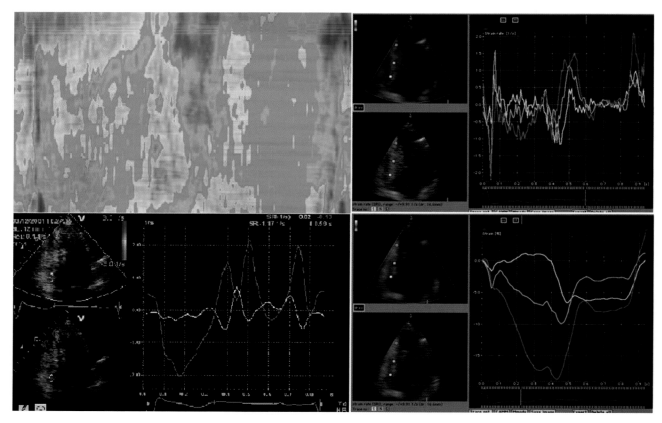

Figure 14.11 Inferior infarction. Top left curved M-mode from apex to base. There is dyskinesia in the basal segment, hypokinesia in the mid-wall segment (the spotted appearance is due to the noise in unfiltered data), and normal shortening in the apex. The two right panels are from the same patient, top strain rate showing the noise in the unfiltered data, while the bottom panel shows the strain curves, demonstrating the smoothing of the integration. Both panels show systolic stretching in the basal segments with post-systolic shortening (yellow trace), reduced shortening with post-systolic shortening in the middle segment (cyan), and normal shortening in the apex (red). For comparison, bottom left shows an inferior infarct from another patient, with akinesia and post-systolic shortening in the base (yellow), and normal strain rate in the apex (blue). This demonstrates the smoothing that is available for strain rate with newer software.

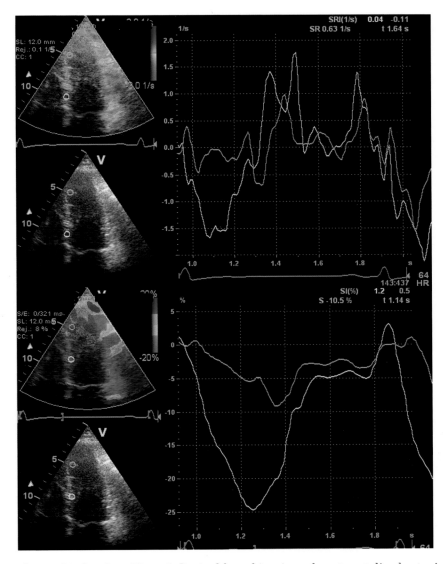

Figure 14.12   Minimal apical infarction. There is limited hypokinesia and post-systolic shortening in the apex. The finding was not apparent in the 2D image, and the initial echo was originally described as normal.

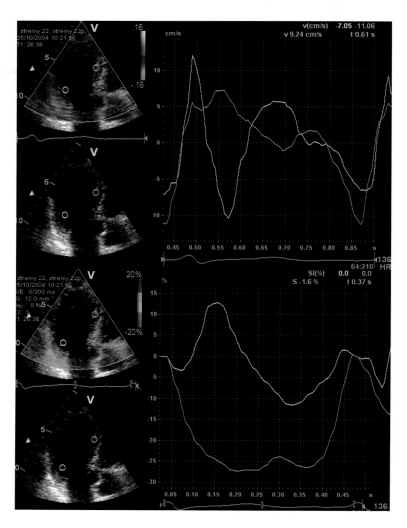

Figure 14.13 Stress echo with apical ischemia. At baseline there is normal systolic shortening, although with a respirational drop out in the apex in the first cycle. At low dose there is increased contractility as evidenced by the increasing red color in systole. At 20 μg there is still normal systolic contractility, but with post-systolic shortening in the apex. At peak stress there is loss of contractility in the apex as well, with increasing post-systolic shortening.

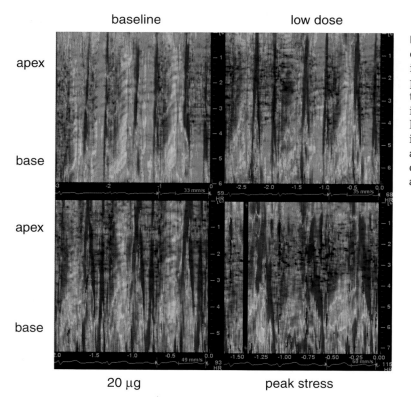

Figure 14.14 Apical long-axis view, stress echo peak stress. The curves show ischemia in the inferolateral wall (yellow trace), compared to fairly normal traces in the anteroseptal wall (cyan). The main finding is a normal isovolumic phase, total dyskinesia in the inferolateral base, and only post-systolic shortening. The anteroseptal wall seems to have an abnormal diastole, but this is due to the fusion of E and A waves as the heart rate is 136, in addition to some diastolic dysfunction.

REFERENCES

1. Heimdal A, Stoylen A, Torp H, Skjaerpe T. Real-time strain rate imaging of the left ventricle by ultrasound. J Am Soc Echocardiogr 1998; 11(11): 1013–19.

2. Amundsen BH, Helle-Valle T, Edvardsen T et al. Noninvasive myocardial strain measurement by speckle tracking echocardiography: validation against sonomicrometry and tagged magnetic resonance imaging. J Am Coll Cardiol 2006; 47(4): 789–93.

3. Leitman M, Lysyansky P, Sidenko S et al. Two-dimensional strain – a novel software for real-time quantitative echocardiographic assessment of myocardial function. J Am Soc Echocardiogr 2004; 17(10): 1021–9.

4. Langeland S, D'hooge J, Wouters PF et al. Experimental validation of a new ultrasound method for the simultaneous assessment of radial and longitudinal myocardial deformation independent of insonation angle. Circulation 2005; 112(14): 2157–62.

5. Fleming AD, Xia X, McDicken WN, Sutherland GR, Fenn L. Myocardial velocity gradients detected by Doppler imaging. Br J Radiol 1994; 67(799): 679–88.

6. Uematsu M, Miyatake K, Tanaka N et al. Myocardial velocity gradient as a new indicator of regional left ventricular contraction: detection by a two-dimensional tissue Doppler imaging technique. J Am Coll Cardiol 1995; 26(1): 217–23.

7. Weidemann F, Jamal F, Sutherland GR et al. Myocardial function defined by strain rate and strain during alterations in inotropic states and heart rate. Am J Physiol Heart Circ Physiol 2002; 283(2): H792–9.

8. Weidemann F, Jamal F, Kowalski M et al. Can strain rate and strain quantify changes in regional systolic function during dobutamine infusion, B-blockade, and atrial pacing – implications for quantitative stress echocardiography. J Am Soc Echocardiogr 2002; 15(5): 416–24.

9. Greenberg NL, Firstenberg MS, Castro PL et al. Doppler-derived myocardial systolic strain rate is a strong index of left ventricular contractility. Circulation 2002; 105(1): 99–105.

10. Cho GY, Chan J, Leano R, Strudwick M, Marwick TH. Comparison of two-dimensional speckle and tissue velocity based strain and validation with harmonic phase magnetic resonance imaging. Am J Cardiol 2006; 97(11): 1661–6.

11. Becker M, Hoffmann R, Kuhl HP et al. Analysis of myocardial deformation based on ultrasonic pixel tracking to determine transmurality in chronic myocardial infarction. Eur Heart J 2006; 27(21): 2560–6.

12. Stoylen A. Strain rate imaging. 2D Strain by speckle tracking. http://folk.ntnu.no/stoylen/strainrate/index.html#2D_strain.

13. Stoylen A, Ingul CB, Torp H. Strain and strain rate parametric imaging. A new method for post processing to 3-/4-dimensional images from three standard apical planes. Preliminary data on feasibility, artefact and regional dyssynergy visualisation. Cardiovasc Ultrasound 2003; 1: 11.

14. Brodin LA, van der Linden J, Olstad B. Echocardiographic functional images based on tissue velocity information. Herz 1998; 23: 1183–99.

15. Stoylen A. Strain rate imaging. Problems, pitfalls and limitations. http://folk.ntnu.no/stoylen/strainrate/Howto/Pitfalls.html.

16. Bohs LN, Trahey GE. A novel method for angle independent ultrasonic imaging of blood flow and tissue motion. IEEE Trans Biomed Eng 1991; 38(3): 280–6.

17. Ingul CB, Torp H, Aase SA et al. Automated analysis of strain rate and strain: feasibility and clinical implications. J Am Soc Echocardiogr 2005; 18(5): 411–18.

18. Sagberg E, Malm S, Ingul CB, Torp H, Støylen A. Feasibility of 3D reconstructed parametric strain rate data in recognition of myocardial infarction. Abstract, Euroecho 8, Athens, 1–4 December 2004. Eur J Echocardiogr 2004; 5(Suppl): S143 (abstract 662).

19. Reisner SA, Lysyansky P, Agmon Y et al. Global longitudinal strain: a novel index of left ventricular systolic function. J Am Soc Echocardiogr 2004; 17(6): 630–3.

20. Eroglu E, Herbots L, Van Cleemput J et al. Ultrasonic strain/strain rate imaging – a new clinical tool to evaluate the transplanted heart. Eur J Echocardiogr 2005; 6(3): 186–95.

21. Simonson JS, Schiller NB. Descent of the base of the left ventricle: an echocardiographic index of left ventricular function. J Am Soc Echocardiogr 1989; 2: 25–35.

22. Gulati VK, Katz WE, Follansbee WP, Gorcsan J 3rd. Mitral annular descent velocity by tissue Doppler echocardiography as an index of global left ventricular function. Am J Cardiol 1996; 77(11): 979–84.

23. Stoylen A, Slordahl S, Skjelvan GK, Heimdal A, Skjaerpe T. Strain rate imaging in normal and reduced diastolic function: comparison with pulsed Doppler tissue imaging of the mitral annulus. J Am Soc Echocardiogr 2001; 14(4): 264–74.

24. Stoylen A, Heimdal A, Bjornstad K, Torp HG, Skjaerpe T. Strain rate imaging by ultrasound in the diagnosis of regional dysfunction of the left ventricle. Echocardiography 1999; 16(4): 321–9.

25. Stoylen A, Heimdal A, Bjornstad K et al. Strain rate imaging by ultrasonography in the diagnosis of coronary artery disease. J Am Soc Echocardiogr 2000; 13(12): 1053–64.

26. Voigt JU, Lindenmeier G, Exner B et al. Incidence and characteristics of segmental postsystolic longitudinal shortening in normal, acutely ischemic, and scarred myocardium. J Am Soc Echocardiogr 2003; 16(5): 415–23.

27. Ingul CB, Stoylen A, Slordahl SA. Recovery of stunned myocardium in acute myocardial infarction quantified by strain rate imaging: a clinical study. J Am Soc Echocardiogr 2005; 18(5): 401–10.

28. Voigt JU, Exner B, Schmiedehausen K et al. Strain-rate imaging during dobutamine stress echocardiography provides objective evidence of inducible ischemia. Circulation 2003; 107(16): 2120–6.

29. Ingul CB, Stoylen A, Slordahl S et al. Automated analysis of myocardial deformation at dobutamine stress echocardiography: an angiographic validation. J Am Coll Cardiol 2007; 49: 1651–9.

15 Cardiac Electrophysiology

Tamas Szili-Torok, Luc J Jordaens and Jos RTC Roelandt

INTRODUCTION

During the last two decades revolutionary diagnostic and therapeutic changes have been implemented in the management of patients with arrhythmias. The development of transcatheter ablation provided a curative treatment of most supraventricular and ventricular tachyarrhythmias. Life-threatening ventricular arrhythmias are effectively palliated by implantable antitachycardia devices and conduction disorders treated by pacemakers, with instantaneous improvement. New challenges are the effective treatment of patients with atrial fibrillation, which is the most frequent and often disabling arrhythmia. Since the arrhythmia substrate is frequently associated with certain anatomic structures or morphologic variants, improved imaging has an increasing role in the improvement of these treatments. Furthermore, novel catheter ablation approaches require catheter placement to sites, which may be associated with an increased risk of complications. Therefore imaging has a crucial role both in guiding and improving the safety of electrophysiology (EP) procedures. In this chapter we discuss how three-dimensional (3D) echocardiography can be used during cardiac EP procedures.

ULTRASOUND SYSTEMS: TECHNICAL BACKGROUND AND APPROACHES

Clinical EP requires invasive procedures since the definitive diagnosis is nearly always made in the EP laboratories immediately followed by curative treatment. This approach requires an imaging technique which can be comfortably used over a long time period without extra cost and personnel. It should increase diagnostic accuracy and decrease the risk for complications. Three-dimensional intracardiac echocardiography (ICE) fulfills most of these criteria.

Two-dimensional intracardiac echocardiography

Recently, two ICE systems became available for interventional EP labs: mechanical and phased-array transducers. The mechanical intravascular ultrasound imaging and ICE system (ClearView, Cardio-Vascular Imaging Systems Inc, Fremont, CA) is an 8 Fr sheath-based catheter that incorporates a 9 MHz beveled single-element transducer rotating at 1800 rpm (model 9900, EP Technologies, Boston Scientific Corp, San Jose, CA, USA).[1] The catheter is equipped with a 1 cm long sonolucent distal sheath with a lumen housing the imaging transducer. The sheath prevents direct contact of the rotating transducer with the cardiac wall. The ICE catheter is filled with 3–5 ml sterile water and then connected to the ultrasound console (model I5007, Boston Scientific Corp, San Jose, CA, USA). This catheter obtains cross-sectional images perpendicular to its long axis. The catheter is relatively simple in its design and the data acquisition allows 3D reconstruction.

The other available system is a 10 Fr catheter-based phased-array transducer operating at 5.5 to 10 MHz frequency and which also has Doppler capabilities (Acuson Corporation, Mountain View, California).[2] The 64-element phased-array transducer allows scanning of a longitudinal 90° sector image with a radial depth penetration of 4 cm. This catheter does not permit 3D reconstruction in its present form. On the other hand, it is a steerable catheter with excellent depth penetration (12 cm), allowing visualization of left-sided structures from the right side of the heart, which is a major advantage in clinical EP.

Three-dimensional echocardiography

Advances in microprocessor technology have made 3D echocardiography a practical imaging modality, providing cardiac structures in realistic forms, which helps to elaborate complex pathology and to reduce interpretation variability. Two different approaches are followed in 3D echocardiography: 3D reconstruction using a sequence of appropriately timed 2D images and real-time volumetric imaging. Currently, automated contour analysis allows measurement and monitoring of global ventricular as well as regional function.

Three-dimensional reconstruction

For 3D reconstructions from intracardiac images, a custom-designed pull-back device for the mechanical ICE transducer is used.[3] This device is controled by the 3D workstation and uses a stepping motor to move the catheter stepwise and linearly in a cephalic–caudal direction through the right atrium. The workstation receives video input from the ICE system and both an ECG and respiration signal (impedance measurement) from the patient (Figure 15.1). Prior to the acquisition run the ranges of RR and breathing intervals are measured to calculate their mean values from the upper and lower limits. Cardiac cycles are recorded and those that

fall within the preset limit (±10%) around the mean interval are further processed. The workstation starts acquisition of 2D images after detecting the peak of the R-wave and in the same phase of respiration, at a speed of 25 images/s (image interval 40 ms), stopping after 1000 ms or after detecting the peak of the R-wave of the next cardiac cycle. After acquiring one cardiac cycle in the preset ranges, the workstation stores the images in the computer main memory, and the catheter is then pulled back by a 0.5 mm axial increment. If the acquired beat falls outside the preset ranges, the ICE transducer is left at the same position and a new cardiac cycle is acquired. This process is repeated until the level of the inferior vena cava (IVC) is reached. Clearly, the acquisition time is much shortened when all cardiac cycles are of the same length. Therefore, in practice the right ventricular apex is paced at 100 bpm. In accordance with their timing in the cardiac cycle, all the individual images of each cardiac cycle are formatted in volumetric datasets (256 × 256 × 256 pixels/each 8 bits) with 40 ms intervals allowing the display of dynamic 3D imaging. During post-processing, several algorithms are applied to reduce noise, enhance edges, and reduce spatial artifacts (ROSA filter).[4]

Real-time volumetric echocardiography

During ICE-guided EP procedures, the EP catheters are continuously manipulated in three dimensions, and the acqusition of the images for 3D reconstruction takes time. Real-time 3D echocardiography, therefore, offers advantages. The Volumetrics® ultrasound system generates real-time 3D pyramidal scanning using a matrix array of 512 crystals. The scanner uses 16 parallel receive channels to generate B-mode images up to 60 volumes per second. Each image plane can be inclined at any desired angle. The LIVE 3D system uses a matrix array with 3000 individual transducers and the system displays

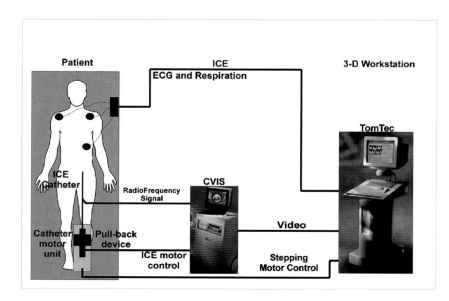

Figure 15.1 Catheterization laboratory setup for three-dimensional reconstruction using an ECG and respiration gated pull-back device.

real-time images.[5] These systems are only for transthoracic use, and prototype systems have been introduced for intracardiac applications. The intracardiac real-time 3D transducer is either incorporated in a 12 Fr catheter and operates at 5 Mhz frequency, or in a 9 Fr catheter and operates at 7 MHz.[6] These catheters were found to be feasible for guiding electrode catheter placement in an open-chest sheep model.[7]

THREE-DIMENSIONAL ECHOCARDIOGRAPHY FOR INTRACARDIAC STRUCTURE IDENTIFICATION

Electrophysiologic mapping and ablation techniques are increasingly used to diagnose and treat many types of supraventricular and ventricular tachycardias. These procedures require an intimate knowledge of intracardiac anatomy and their use has led to a renewed interest in visualization of specific structures. Classical imaging techniques may be unable to visualize structures involved in arrhythmia mechanisms and therapy. This part of the chapter provides electrophysiologists with an overview of recent insights into the structure of the heart obtained with 3D intracardiac echocardiography and indicates to the echo-specialist which structures are potentially important for the electrophysiologist.

The interatrial septum (Figure 15.2)

Anatomically and echocardiographically the most prominent part of the atria is the interatrial septum with its very characteristic appearance. It is defined as the thin wall separating the two atria, running obliquely from the front, extending posteriorly and to the right. When it is seen from the right atrium, the most prominent feature is the fossa ovalis surrounded by a muscular rim. When seen from the left atrium, the crater-like appearance of the right side

is absent. The membrane in the fossa itself is predominantly composed of fibrous tissue with relatively few myocytes. Although the interatrial septum was a focus of interest for congenital disorders, electrophysiologists have discovered additional reasons to explore the interatrial septum. A significant number of accessory pathways are located septally. Their close relation to the natural atrioventricular conduction system means that direct visualization of the septum can theoretically improve the safety of ablation procedures. Furthermore, left atrioventricular accessory pathways can be approached using the transseptal approach, which provides improved stability for the ablation catheter. This requires puncture of the interatrial septum. Although it can be done without direct imaging, data clearly demonstrate improved safety and increased efficacy using intracardiac echocardiography.[8,9] Another important electrophysiologic aspect of the interatrial septum is related to the natural conduction pathways between the two atria. These special fibers are located both anteriorly above the fossa ovalis and posteriorly near the orifice of the coronary sinus. Recent data suggest that interatrial conduction delay may play a significant role in the onset mechanism of atrial fibrillation.[10]

Coronary sinus (Figure 15.3)

The coronary sinus (CS) is a small tubular structure just above the posterior left atrioventricular junction. The CS is of special interest to the electrophysiologist and pacemaker-implanting physician. It opens into the right atrium between the inferior vena cava and the tricuspid valve orifice. Its tributaries are the great, small, and middle cardiac veins, the posterior vein of the left ventricle, and the oblique vein of the left atrium (Marshall's vein), all except the last having valves at their orifices. Left atrial recording for EP studies is routinely done indirectly from the CS. The left atrium or the left ventricle can also be paced via the CS. The CS can be cannulated from the jugular, subclavian, or femoral vein

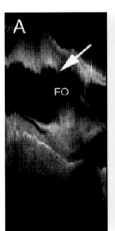
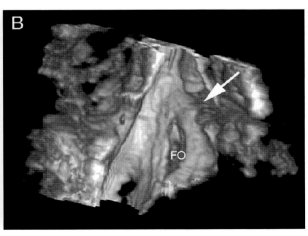

Figure 15.2 A) "En face" view of the interatrial septum with the oval fossa. B) reconstruction of the right atrium from a volumetric data set. The arrows indicate the Bachmann's bundle region of the interatrial septum.

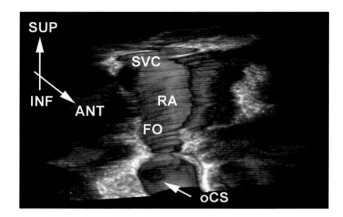

Figure 15.3 Three-dimensional echocardiographic *en face* view of the ostium of coronary sinus. RA, right atrium; AWT, anterior; INF, inferior; CS, coronary sinus; FO, oval fossa; SVC, superior caval vein.

and insertion of pacing/diagnostic electrode catheters is easy in most patients. However, in some patients cannulation of the CS or its tributaries can pose significant difficulties and may result in excessive procedural and fluoroscopy time. Theoretically 3D ICE can identify anatomic variants and may facilitate such procedures.[11] Apart from its obvious role in providing access to the left atrioventricular junction during EP testing, the CS is an important structure for the electrophysiologist.

Resynchronization by simultaneous electrical stimulation of both ventricles significantly improves hemodynamics, resulting in increased exercise tolerance and hence quality of life in patients with advanced heart failure and intraventricular conduction delay.[12] This simultaneous stimulation is achieved by positioning the left ventricular electrode through the CS into its left ventricular side branches. Furthermore, biatrial stimulation was also reportedly effective in the preventive treatment of patients with paroxysmal atrial fibrillation.[10]

Valves in the coronary sinus (Figure 15.4)

In the majority of cases the great cardiac vein possesses a prominent valve where the vein turns around the obtuse margin to become the coronary sinus. This valve was first described by the French scientist R. Vieussens in his book *Nouvelles découvertes sur le coeur* (Paris, 1706). Until recently, all of these anatomic variants are known from postmortem human studies. A certain level of anecdotal relationship is proposed between difficulties during interventions in cardiac electrophysiology and anatomic differences, but there has been no systematically conducted study to provide direct evidence. One of the reasons is that fluoroscopy – which is an almost exclusive tool for guiding EP procedures – does not allow visualization of anatomic landmarks.

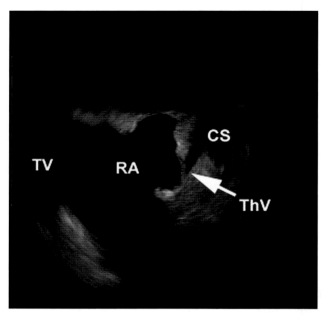

Figure 15.4 Horizontal cross-sectional intracardiac echocardiography image with a valve in the ostium of the coronary sinus. CS, coronary sinus; RAA, right atrial appendage; ThV, thebesian valve; TV, tricuspid valve.

Eustachian ridge and valve and the Thebesian valve (Figure 15.5)

The right and left venous valves of the sino-atrial orifice regulate the flow of blood from the sinus venosus to the atrium in fish, amphibians, and reptiles. In birds, mammals, and humans, the venous valve loses its hemodynamic function and only comes to medical attention when congenital anomalies occur that are related to it.[13] The right venous valve persists in humans as the crista terminalis, Eustachian, and Thebesian valves. An intraluminal muscle band has been described located inside the right atrium, and coursing in the line of the crista terminalis between the septum spurium and inferior vena cava. This abnormality is possibly derived from the right venous valve. Usually it has a triangular shape and is a flap of fibrous fibro-muscular tissue that is inserted on the Eustachian ridge. The Eustachian ridge separates the orifices of the inferior caval vein and CS. In some cases the valve is particularly large and can be an obstacle to catheters passing from the inferior caval vein. Occasionally the valve is perforated or takes the form of delicate filigreed mesh. The free border of the valve is called the tendon of Todaro. This tendon runs in the musculature of the sinus septum. This is indeed one of the borders of Koch's triangle. The detailed information and clinical significance of the Eustachian valve have not yet been elucidated. In the cases of atrial fibrillation with severe tricuspid regurgitation, the valve remains at the semi-closed position throughout systole and opened in the rapid filling phase. A small crescentic flap, the Thebesian valve, usually guards the orifice of the coronary sinus. Frequently it is fenestrated. An imperforate valve completely covering the ostium is very rare, but can be a major obstacle for positioning electrode catheters into the CS.

Koch's triangle (Figure 15.6)

The structures delaying the cardiac impulse and then insuring its rapid propagation to the ventricular myocardium constitute a continuous axis of histologically discrete cells. The atrial components are located at the base of the atrial septum, located at the apex of a triangular region first illustrated by Koch. The anterior border is marked by the hinge of the septal leaflet of the tricuspid valve. Superiorly,

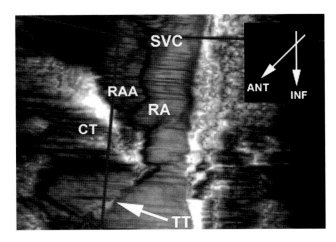

Figure 15.5 The tendon of Todaro reconstructed from a 3D dataset. CT, terminal crest; ANT, anterior; INF, inferior; RA, right atrium; SVC, superior caval vein; TT, tendon of Todaro.

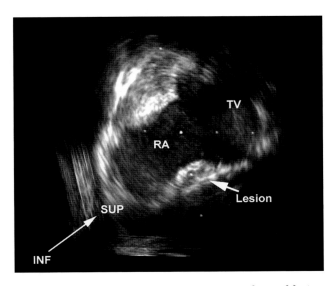

Figure 15.6 *En face* 3D reconstruction of an ablation lesion visualized as low contrast area in human Koch's triangle using 3D myocardial contrast echocardiography. INF, inferior; RA, right atrium; TV, tricuspid valve.

the central fibrous body is the landmark for penetration of the bundle of His. The inferior border of the triangle is the orifice of the CS and the vestibule immediately anterior to it. This part is the area which is targeted for ablation of the slow pathway in atrio-ventricular nodal re-entrant tachycardia (AVNRT). The so-called fast pathway corresponds to the area of musculature close to the apex of the triangle. Ablation in Koch's triangle was of special interest in the last two decades. A large number of patients with supraventricular tachycardia have an AVNRT. The occurrence of inadvertent complete AV block is an infrequent but serious complication.[14] Imaging of this region using ICE is not particularly difficult, because of the very characteristic appearance of the borders. Intracardiac ultrasound was reported during AVNRT ablation to improve the outcome of the procedures. During cryo-ablation of the AV node the cryocatheter–endocardial contact and ice-ball growth could be effectively monitored with ICE.[15]

THREE-DIMENSIONAL ECHOCARDIOGRAPHY FOR GUIDING ELECTROPHYSIOLOGY PROCEDURES

Transthoracic echocardiography has several limitations during interventions. It requires additional trained personnel and violation of sterility is a major problem. Transesophageal echocardiography (TEE) is potentially useful, and provides superior images for intracardiac structure identification. The major problem with this technique is the need for general anesthesia, since EP procedures are often complex and lengthy which may result in significant patient discomfort. Recently ICE became available, providing excellent accuracy in direct visualization of anatomic landmarks.

Transseptal puncture

Percutaneous puncture of the interatrial septum was introduced for catheterization of the left heart in 1960.[16] Recently there has been renewed interest in transseptal left heart catheterization due to the development of left-sided catheter ablations.[17–20] However, a significant number of acute and potentially lethal complications with transseptal puncture may occur, including tamponade, systemic emboli, and even death secondary to aortic perforation.[17,20] The conventional technique relies on fluoroscopic landmarks to define anatomic boundaries and detection of the movement of the tip of the device from the thicker muscular septum to the thin wall of the fossa ovalis. Since fluoroscopy does not allow direct visualization of the fossa ovalis, transseptal catheterization remains a difficult procedure, particularly in the cases where the atrial anatomy is atypical. Therefore imaging techniques such as TEE and 2D transthoracic echocardiography have been used for the assessment of the interatrial septum during transseptal puncture.[21–26] Both techniques have limitations. Transthoracic ultrasound may not be able to accurately locate the thin wall of the fossa ovalis. Furthermore, transthoracic echocardiography is fairly uncomfortable to perform without a risk of violation of sterility during the intervention. TEE is an alternative method but causes lengthening of the procedure because of the introduction of the esophageal probe, and because it requires intravenous sedation for a longer period, limits the communication with the patient during the procedure, and needs an experienced operator. Intracardiac ultrasound allows visualization of the fossa ovalis in all patients with excellent image quality.[27–30] This is a direct method and a possible means to avoid complications. In recent studies, in which patients underwent transseptal puncture under ICE guidance, the success rate was always higher than with fluoroscopy and there were no complications.[8,9] In our institute we always confirm the success of the puncture by a contrast injection through the Brockenbrough needle and its appearance in the left atrium detected by ICE.[8,31]

Inappropriate sinus tachycardia

The technique for ablative modification of sinus node function guided by ICE has been extensively described in animals and humans.[32–34] At present there are no clear guidelines to describe which patients should undergo such a procedure, as the recurrence rate remains fairly high. Moreover, it seems that patients undergoing multiple sinus node modification procedures are at higher risk for superior vena cava syndrome.[33,35] CARTO mapping has a potential to guide this procedure, but the method is indirect and the advantage of continuous monitoring of the diameter of the vena cava superior is lost.[36]

Atrial tachycardia

Atrial tachycardias originate from specific identifiable anatomic structures that are not seen on fluoroscopy. Crista terminalis in the right atrium and the pulmonary veins in the left atrium are most frequently involved. Kalman and colleagues have demonstrated that approximately two-thirds of focal right atrial tachycardias in patients without structural heart disease arise along the crista terminalis. Direct visualization of these structures undoubtedly facilitates mapping and ablation of these tachycardias.[11]

Atrial flutter

Atrial flutter (AFL) is a frequent arrhythmia due to re-entry around the large vascular structures in the right atrium.[37,38] ICE is an excellent imaging tool to clarify the anatomy of the cavo-tricuspid isthmus and its variations, which is a slow conducting zone of the macrore-entry circuit.[39–41] Because the maneuverability of the mechanical transducer is limited it is difficult to optimally visualize the isthmus and the adjacent intracardiac structures.[28] In these cases introduction of the ICE catheter through the subclavian vein is helpful.[28] By the use of phased-array and steerable probes this problem seems to be overcome.[42] In flutter ablation ICE also has a role to identify anatomic obstacles such as the Eustachian ridge, Thebesian vein, and the tricuspid annulus, and the catheter–wall contact can be appropriately monitored.

Linear ablations for the treatment of atrial fibrillation

Recently, attempts have been made to treat atrial fibrillation by creating multiple linear atrial lesions with RF energy. ICE offers imaging of endocardial anatomy and the ablation electrode–tissue interface, which is not available with standard fluoroscopy. Compared with fluoroscopy, ICE guidance has been shown to improve targeting, energy delivery, and lesion formation and to prevent energy delivery to potentially dangerous sites in a canine model.[43] ICE also demonstrates significant sliding of the catheter despite apparent catheter stability assessed by electrograms.[44,45]

Pulmonary vein ablation for atrial fibrillation

Atrial fibrillation can be initiated by triggers originating from various sites in the atria. However, the origin of the triggers lies in the atrial tissue extending in the pulmonary veins. Correct identification of the anatomy is important since significant variations exist, including a common vestibule of the left pulmonary veins and additional small branches. ICE has a critically important role in ablation in this region. First, the transseptal puncture can be guided by ICE. Pulmonary venous anatomy can be assessed using the phased-array transducer without entering the left side of the heart. During ablation the wall contact of the catheters can be monitored. In view of the fact that pulmonary vein stenosis is the most frequent and potentially life-threatening complication of the procedure,[46] one of the major advantages of ICE appears to be that after ablation pulmonary vein stenosis can be reliably assessed using vessel diameter measurement and Doppler flow measurements. Reports suggest that pulmonary venous anatomy can be extensively studied by 3D ICE, including visualization of ablation catheters in the vein.[47,48]

Ventricular tachycardia

In general, association of structural abnormalities and arrhythmogenesis can be confirmed with ICE.

The site of origin of idiopathic ventricular tachycardia (VT) arising from the left ventricular outflow tract (LVOT) may be closely related to the aortic valve leaflets, and radiofrequency (RF) delivery potentially can damage them. Idiopathic VT of the LVOT can be treated successfully with RF ablation. ICE can identify accurately the ablation electrode and the anatomic landmarks while the contact with the endocardium is easily assessed.[49] Scar-related ventricular tachycardias could also be mapped with the assistance of ICE by identifying scar tissue and adjacent isthmuses of viable tissue.

Ablation in the region of Koch's triangle

AV nodal re-entry tachycardias and AV nodes are successfully ablated in more than 97% of patients, suggesting that imaging is not particularly necessary for these ablations. On the other hand, testing novel ablation approaches such as cryothermy can be performed under echocardiographic monitoring. During cryoablation of the AV node the cryocatheter–endocardial contact and iceball growth can be effectively monitored with ICE.[15]

Assessment of ablation lesions (Figure 15.6)

Tissue changes could be theoretically detected by ICE. Crater formation and increased echodensity were reported immediately after RF ablation.[34] However, we could not see RF lesions 20 minutes after ablation.[28] Therefore, local wall thickness was studied as an indirect sign and has some relation with the lesion size, although this is insufficient to make intra-procedural decisions.[50] There is a need for direct visualization of the ablation of such lesions. Myocardial contrast echocardiography together with ICE is currently being studied to directly visualize RF lesions after focal and linear ablation. This method can be combined with a 3D reconstruction technique.[51]

Guiding pacing procedures: pacemaker implantation without the use of fluoroscopy?

Echocardiography has been used to guide temporary electrode catheter insertion in the emergency room and intensive care setting when fluoroscopy is not promptly available. Pacemaker implantations were guided by TEE during the first trimester of pregnancy in patients with second-degree heart block and syncope. TEE was found to be very appropriate to confirm satisfactory electrode position in the right atrial appendage.[52,53] Recently, novel ways of pacing have been proposed for the treatment of patients with various types of arrhythmias.[35,54,55] There is growing evidence suggesting that pacing on the atrial level in the region of Bachmann's bundle, the interatrial septum, or even multiple atrial sites may have advantages in patients with atrial

fibrillation.[10,54,55] On the ventricular level, novel pacing techniques may have a role in preserving or even improving ventricular performance in patients with or without heart failure.[12] However, these specific site pacing techniques require an extremely accurate lead positioning as compared to the conventional bradycardia indications. This may explain that adequate results are not obtained with these new pacing therapies in a considerable number of patients. One of the explanations is possibly related to the anatomic variations resulting in a variable and less efficient lead positioning. We developed and tested a novel technique based on 3D ICE for specific site pacing[56] (Figures 15.7 and 15.8).

Monitoring of potential complications (Figure 15.9)

A potential complication of all EP procedures is the development of pericardial fluid and pericardial

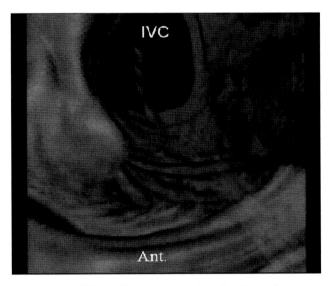

Figure 15.7 Three-dimensional visualization of a pacemaker electrode in the right atrium. Ant, anterior; IVC, inferior caval vein.

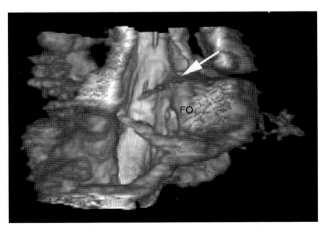

Figure 15.8 Bachmann's bundle pacing could be achieved with 3D echocardiography guiding. FO, oval fossa.

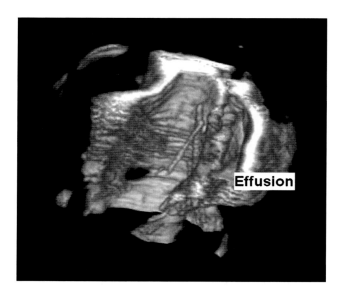

Figure 15.9 Pericardial effusion detected with 3D echocardiography.

tamponade. Continuous monitoring using echocardiography has the potential to detect this at a very early stage and therefore appropriate treatment can be applied.

CONCLUSIONS

Two basic directions of the development of ultrasound imaging have been seen in recent decades: miniaturization and 3D imaging. Clinical EP has significantly benefited from both directions allowing the use of intracardiac transducers and 3D imaging for better intracardiac structure identification. The application of these current devices in clinical EP is the focus of ongoing research. When real-time 3D echocardiography becomes routinely available, EP and pacing procedures can be guided with improved safety and accuracy, with further reduction in the use of fluoroscopy. This will be a major asset for imaging and interventional cardiac EP.

REFERENCES

1. Chu E, Fitzpatrick AP, Chin MC et al. Radiofrequency catheter ablation guided by intracardiac echocardiography. Circulation 1994; 89: 1301–5.

2. Bruce CJ, Packer DL, Seward JB. Intracardiac Doppler hemodynamics and flow: new vector, phased-array ultrasound-tipped catheter. Am J Cardiol 1999; 83: 1509–12, A9.

3. Roelandt JR, di Mario C, Pandian NG et al. Three-dimensional reconstruction of intracoronary ultrasound images. Rationale, approaches, problems, and directions. Circulation 1994; 90: 1044–55.

4. Bruining N, von Birgelen C, Di Mario C. Dynamic three-dimensional reconstruction of ICUS images on an ECG-gated pull-back device. In: Press ICS, ed. Computers in Cardiology. Vienna: IEEE Computer Society Press, 1995.

5. von Ramm O, Smith S. Real-time volumetric ultrasound imaging system. J Digit Imaging 1990; 3: 261–6.

6. Light ED, Idriss SF, Wolf PD, Smith SW. Real-time three-dimensional intracardiac echocardiography. Ultrasound Med Biol 2001; 27: 1177–83.

7. Smith SW, Light ED, Idriss SF, Wolf PD. Feasibility study of real-time three-dimensional intracardiac echocardiography for guidance of interventional electrophysiology. Pacing Clin Electrophysiol 2002; 25: 351–7.

8. Szili-Torok T, Kimman G, Theuns D et al. Transseptal left heart catheterisation guided by intracardiac echocardiography. Heart 2001; 86: E11.

9. Daoud EG, Kalbfleisch SJ, Hummel JD. Intracardiac echocardiography to guide transseptal left heart catheterization for radiofrequency catheter ablation. J Cardiovasc Electrophysiol 1999; 10: 358–63.

10. Saksena S, Delfaut P, Prakash A, Kaushik RR, Krol RB. Multisite electrode pacing for prevention of atrial fibrillation. J Cardiovasc Electrophysiol 1998; 9: S155–62.

11. Kalman JM, Olgin JE, Karch MR et al. 'Cristal tachycardias': origin of right atrial tachycardias from the crista terminalis identified by intracardiac echocardiography. J Am Coll Cardiol 1998; 31: 451–9.

12. Cazeau S, Leclercq C, Lavergne T et al. Effects of multisite biventricular pacing in patients with heart failure and intraventricular conduction delay. N Engl J Med 2001; 344: 873–80.

13. Ansalone G, Giannantoni P, Ricci R et al. Doppler myocardial imaging to evaluate the effectiveness of pacing sites in patients receiving biventricular pacing. J Am Coll Cardiol 2002; 39: 489–99.

14. Scheinman MM, Huang S. The 1998 NASPE prospective catheter ablation registry. Pacing Clin Electrophysiol 2000; 23: 1020–8.

15. Dubuc M, Khairy P, Rodriguez-Santiago A et al. Catheter cryoablation of the atrioventricular node in patients with atrial fibrillation: a novel technology for ablation of cardiac arrhythmias. J Cardiovasc Electrophysiol 2001; 12: 439–44.

16. Brockenbrough E, Braunwald E. A new technique for left ventricular angiography and transseptal left heart catheterization. Am J Cardiol 1960; 6: 1062–7.

17. Blomstrom-Lundqvist C, Olsson SB, Varnauskas E. Transseptal left heart catheterization: a review of 278 studies. Clin Cardiol 1986; 9: 21–6.

18. Lesh MD, Van Hare GF, Scheinman MM, Ports TA, Epstein LA. Comparison of the retrograde and transseptal methods for ablation of left free wall accessory pathways. J Am Coll Cardiol 1993; 22: 542–9.

19. Montenero AS, Crea F, Bendini MG, Bellocci F, Zecchi P. Catheter ablation of left accessory atrioventricular connections: the transseptal approach. J Interven Cardiol 1995; 8: 806–12.

20. Roelke M, Smith AJ, Palacios IF. The technique and safety of transseptal left heart catheterization: the Massachusetts General Hospital experience with 1,279 procedures. Cathet Cardiovasc Diagn 1994; 32: 332–9.

21. Hurrell DG, Nishimura RA, Symanski JD, Holmes DR Jr. Echocardiography in the invasive laboratory: utility of

two-dimensional echocardiography in performing transseptal catheterization. Mayo Clin Proc 1998; 73: 126–31.

22. Hahn K, Bajwa T, Sarnoski J, Schmidt DH, Gal R. Transseptal catheterization with transesophageal guidance in high risk patients. Echocardiography 1997; 14: 475–80.

23. Hahn K, Gal R, Sarnoski J et al. Transesophageal echocardiographically guided atrial transseptal catheterization in patients with normal-sized atria: incidence of complications. Clin Cardiol 1995; 18: 217–20.

24. Kantoch MJ, Frost GF, Robertson MA. Use of transesophageal echocardiography in radiofrequency catheter ablation in children and adolescents. Can J Cardiol 1998; 14: 519–23.

25. Tucker KJ, Curtis AB, Murphy J et al. Transesophageal echocardiographic guidance of transseptal left heart catheterization during radiofrequency ablation of left-sided accessory pathways in humans. Pacing Clin Electrophysiol 1996; 19: 272–81.

26. Kyo S, Motoyama T, Miyamoto N et al. Percutaneous introduction of left atrial cannula for left heart bypass: utility of biplane transesophageal echocardiographic guidance for transseptal puncture. Artif Organs 1992; 16: 386–91.

27. Epstein LM. The utility of intracardiac echocardiography in interventional electrophysiology. Curr Cardiol Rep 2000; 2: 329–34.

28. Szili-Torok T, Kimman G, Theuns D et al. Visualisation of intracardiac structures and radiofrequency lesions using intracardiac echocardiography. Eur J Echocardiogr 2003; 4: 17–22.

29. Foster GP, Picard MH. Intracardiac echocardiography: current uses and future directions. Echocardiography 2001; 18: 43–8.

30. Kalman JM, Olgin JE, Karch MR, Lesh MD. Use of intracardiac echocardiography in interventional electrophysiology. Pacing Clin Electrophysiol 1997; 20: 2248–62.

31. Szili-Torok T, Kimman GJ, Tuin J, Jordaens L. How to approach left-sided accessory pathway ablation using intracardiac echocardiography. Europace 2001; 3: 28.

32. Kalman JM, Lee RJ, Fisher WG et al. Radiofrequency catheter modification of sinus pacemaker function guided by intracardiac echocardiography. Circulation 1995; 92: 3070–81.

33. Lee RJ, Kalman JM, Fitzpatrick AP et al. Radiofrequency catheter modification of the sinus node for 'inappropriate' sinus tachycardia. Circulation 1995; 92: 2919–28.

34. Ren JF, Marchlinski FE, Callans DJ, Zado ES. Echocardiographic lesion characteristics associated with successful ablation of inappropriate sinus tachycardia. J Cardiovasc Electrophysiol 2001; 12: 814–18.

35. Callans DJ, Ren JF, Schwartzman D et al. Narrowing of the superior vena cava–right atrium junction during radiofrequency catheter ablation for inappropriate sinus tachycardia: analysis with intracardiac echocardiography. J Am Coll Cardiol 1999; 33: 1667–70.

36. Leonelli F, Richey M, Beheiry S, Rajkovich K, Natale A. Tridimensional mapping: guided modification of the sinus node. J Cardiovasc Electrophysiol 1998; 9: 1214–17.

37. Cosio FG, Lopez-Gil M, Goicolea A, Arribas F. Electrophysiologic studies in atrial flutter. Clin Cardiol 1992; 15: 667–73.

38. Klein GJ, Guiraudon GM, Sharma AD, Milstein S. Demonstration of macroreentry and feasibility of operative therapy

in the common type of atrial flutter. Am J Cardiol 1986; 57: 587–91.

39. Friedman PA, Luria D, Fenton AM et al. Global right atrial mapping of human atrial flutter: the presence of postero-medial (sinus venosa region) functional block and double potentials: a study in biplane fluoroscopy and intracardiac echocardiography. Circulation 2000; 101: 1568–77.

40. Lesh MD, Kalman JM, Karch MR. Use of intracardiac echocardiography during electrophysiologic evaluation and therapy of atrial arrhythmias. J Cardiovasc Electrophysiol 1998; 9: S40–7.

41. Olgin JE, Kalman JM, Fitzpatrick AP, Lesh MD. Role of right atrial endocardial structures as barriers to conduction during human type I atrial flutter. Activation and entrainment mapping guided by intracardiac echocardiography. Circulation 1995; 92: 1839–48.

42. Morton JB, Sanders P, Byrne MJ et al. Phased-array intracardiac echocardiography to guide radiofrequency ablation in the left atrium and at the pulmonary vein ostium. J Cardiovasc Electrophysiol 2001; 12: 343–8.

43. Epstein LM, Mitchell MA, Smith TW, Haines DE. Comparative study of fluoroscopy and intracardiac echocardiographic guidance for the creation of linear atrial lesions. Circulation 1998; 98: 1796–801.

44. Chu E, Kalman JM, Kwasman MA et al. Intracardiac echocardiography during radiofrequency catheter ablation of cardiac arrhythmias in humans. J Am Coll Cardiol 1994; 24: 1351–7.

45. Scholten M, Szili-Torok T, Kimman G et al. Right atrial linear ablation for paroxysmal AF guided by intracardiac echocardiography. Thoraxcentre J 2002; 14/1: 27–9.

46. Gerstenfeld EP, Guerra P, Sparks PB, Hattori K, Lesh MD. Clinical outcome after radiofrequency catheter ablation of focal atrial fibrillation triggers. J Cardiovasc Electrophysiol 2001; 12: 900–8.

47. Schwartzmann D, Panescu D, Lardner R. Full-motion, three-dimensional pulmonary vein imaging using intracardiac echocardiography. Pacing Clin Electrophysiol 2002; 24: 617.

48. Simon R. Use of three-dimensional intracardiac echocardiography for assessment of pulmonary vein anatomy and Lasso catheter localization. J Am Coll Cardiol 2002; 39(Suppl A): 349A.

49. Lamberti F, Calo L, Pandozi C et al. Radiofrequency catheter ablation of idiopathic left ventricular outflow tract tachycardia: utility of intracardiac echocardiography. J Cardiovasc Electrophysiol 2001; 12: 529–35.

50. Ren JF, Callans DJ, Schwartzman D, Michele JJ, Marchlinski FE. Changes in local wall thickness correlate with pathologic lesion size following radiofrequency catheter ablation: an intracardiac echocardiographic imaging study. Echocardiography 2001; 18: 503–7.

51. Khoury D, Rao L, Panescu D. Reconstruction of linear ablation lesions by three-dimensional myocardial contrast echocardiography. Pacing Clin Electrophysiol 2002; 24: 640.

52. Jordaens LJ, Vandenbogaerde JF, Van de Bruaene P, De Buyzere M. Transesophageal echocardiography for insertion of a physiological pacemaker in early pregnancy. Pacing Clin Electrophysiol 1990; 13: 955–7.

53. Antonelli D, Bloch L, Rosenfeld T. Implantation of permanent dual chamber pacemaker in a pregnant woman by transesophageal echocardiographic guidance. Pacing Clin Electrophysiol 1999; 22: 534–5.

54. Bailin SJ, Adler S, Giudici M. Prevention of chronic atrial fibrillation by pacing in the region of Bachmann's

bundle: results of a multicenter randomized trial. J Cardiovasc Electrophysiol 2001; 12: 912–17.

55. Padeletti L, Pieragnoli P, Ciapetti C et al. Randomized crossover comparison of right atrial appendage pacing versus interatrial septum pacing for prevention of paroxysmal atrial fibrillation in patients with sinus bradycardia. Am Heart J 2001; 142: 1047–55.

56. Szili-Torok T, Scholten M, Ligthart J et al. Interatrial septum pacing guided by three-dimensional intracardiac echocardiography. J Am Coll Cardiol 2002; 39(Suppl): 99A.

Index

(Page numbers in italics refer to figures and tables)